And Then Again...

by

Ron Stewart

Published by New Generation Publishing in 2012

Copyright © Ron Stewart 2012

First Edition

www.newgeneration-publishing.com

 **New Generation Publishing**

All ideas, memories, thoughts and emotions in this book are the domain of Ron Stewart.

The book is his work as a tribute to all those who fight against cancer, either because it has attacked their bodies, or because they have committed themselves professionally to help those in that position.

This is a story based on Ron's experience. It is one of many millions. There may be some similarities but everyone is an individual experience.

"All that is necessary for Evil to triumph is for good men to do nothing."

Commonly attributed to Edmund Burke (1729-1797) but probably incorrectly.

"But the wicked are like the troubled sea, when it cannot rest, whose waters cast up mire and dirt."

Isaiah, chapter 57:20

1

The air exploded from my body with a force that took me by surprise. Never in all my years of back alley fights and violent arrests had I been left so winded by a blow. Never in all my years of playing contact sports had anyone ever hit me so hard as to make me feel this way.

My body hung forward, shoulders slack. My jaw open I realised air was coming back down my throat in short, sharp breaths. Squeezing my eyes shut to help gain some form of self control I was assailed by a galaxy of colours taking me down a swirling spiral. In a brief second of rational, if dislocated, thought I realised the colours reminded me of the weather maps of my school days long ago: red for the intense heat of deserts indicating wild panic; orange for hot climes, but more manageable; moving into green for temperate circumstances. It would have been so comforting to stay there but the rush down and round continued: Mediterranean blue for cooler climes and the chill that was enveloping me, before arriving at the blue tinged white of Arctic ice and the cold fear that that now gripped me.

My breathing steadied. I realised that no-one had hit me. There had been no physical violence against me. All that had happened was the other man in the room with me had just spoken three words.

I raised my head and looked at that man who was courteously, and discreetly, polishing his spectacles. His brown skin and features gave every clue as to his origins on the Indian sub-continent. His white coat and stethoscope gave every clue to his profession.

"Doctor, could you say that again, please?"

"Of course. I said you have cancer."

2

Eight months later I sat in the office on a beautiful May afternoon contemplating going home. I had been back at work on a regular basis for one week. My superiors had been very understanding. I was just doing day work for the time being, nothing too demanding. Tasked by my Detective Inspector I was doing crime reviews, including a lot of time watching CCTV footage. I didn't mind that. I had lots of experience of watching things.

As I mused over the options on going home I realised that I had started to contemplate ideas on where I might stop off for a light refreshment. It was warm and the possibility of a long, cool glass of lager had a certain appeal.

Even that thought made me feel better. Just as recently as a month earlier the mere thought of such a drink would have caused me to wretch. A month before I was as bald as the proverbial billiard ball. Now my head had a covering of hair like fine down and I had been concerned to note the need to shave once a week or so. After months of total economy on shaving razors that development would cause havoc with my budget !

My mind wandered back over the past months. From initial misgivings and concerns to full diagnosis and the wild fluctuations of physical and emotional reaction to the treatment. It had been one hell of a journey but whether it had been slow or fast was difficult to decide.

My mind drifted once more, as it had many times over the immediate past months, over the question of why it happened to me. Getting cancer is what happened to other people. There was no reason to think I would ever get it. I had not even felt ill when the whole business started on its crazy journey. In fact, I had felt fine.

I had often wondered about the how and why. There had been many questions into my life style, physical injuries. So many questions over whether I had been kicked in my private parts. In my profession, and sporting activity it had been so easy to reply in the affirmative, but that had been a few years in the past.

It had caused me to look back over my life and review its direction. I had lost track of the times I had come to crossroads of life and chosen the next direction. If at any, or many, of those crossroads had I chosen differently would it have saved me from cancer, I wondered. The answer was as transparent to me as a politician playing poker.

There was absolutely no way of knowing.

Yet still I reviewed the possibilities. Perhaps that was just the policeman in me. There had to be clues that fitted together to give me the answer, but somehow the investigation was at a level that was beyond me, and my energy levels. If I could just accept that even the medical world could not identify what initiated cancer I may just have an easier mind about it.

My mind wandered further back into my life. I was born in Lossiemouth, Morayshire, Scotland, which had its easiest reference point as the home of Ramsay McDonald, first Labour Prime Minister. My father had worked at the Royal Naval Air Station following his wartime service with the RAF. Perhaps that was the first clue as to some form of deviation. Up until then all of his father's family had been fishermen, but my dad chose otherwise. Maybe if he had done differently it would have all have worked out otherwise. Not going on the boats had created other opportunities. My old man had been such a promising golfer he had been offered the chance to become a professional, but in the

7

1930's that was a very precarious option, and provided none of the inducements of modern times. Instead he had taken a trade to ensure his livelihood.

That trade took the family the length and breadth of the country in the service of the crown. It also took us to other parts of the world. Perhaps something happened to my body when I was abroad and it had just lain dormant for all those years.

On leaving school I had followed my father into the Ministry of Defence and started work in London. I enjoyed it to a point: but not enough. After a couple of years I left to do what I had always felt was for me, and joined the Metropolitan Police.

Apart from an unhappy marriage, which was fortuitously brief, with no issue as a constant reminder, the following years had been an intoxicating mix of excitement, camaraderie and advancement. Time in the Special Patrol Group and Drug Squad had given me all the adrenalin rushes I would ever need.

That was until the fateful day I had lost my best friend. The thought jolted me from my reverie. My life had been a roller coaster. The past few months had been that way, as well. I started to drift off thinking about those months when the building shuddered with the effects of an explosion.

The colours danced and spiralled before my eyes again. Red to orange to blue to ice blue white. Fear gripped me . That was not just an explosion: that was a bomb.

The time was 4.20 p.m.

3

"Right, tonight's the night. You've all had your pre briefings. There will be three teams, each with uniformed support."

Detective Inspector Sam Mitchell was in charge of Operation Sister Sledge. For months the gang of Kosovans had been tracked and evidence painstakingly gathered. Drugs, prostitution, people trafficking and the odd bit of gun running were all activities that had been duly noted.

The team has gathered at the nearest station to the target in the Canary Wharf area. There had been a significant influx of immigrants from the Balkans over to escape the atrocities of the old Yugoslavia. Opportunists had seen the chance of a good life for themselves, even if it only meant a different misery for others.

Some of the local elements had taken exception to the invasion of their home area, and word soon filtered through to the police. Circumstances always created strange alliances.

Pointing to a layout plan hanging from the wall the DI continued "Team A will take the front entrance. Teams B and C will seal off the east and west wing entrances. The target flat is on the first floor immediately above the main entrance. Team A will only enter when B and C are in position closing off all other exits."

Barry nudged me and gave me a conspiratorial wink. We were both in Team A. Both of us has taken part in similar raids and become more than expert in the art of quick entry and apprehensions. We had adopted an unofficial practice of alternating the lead. Tonight it was my turn to go in first.

The convoy of cars and vans swung into position

with no fanfare, sealing off the car parks to the flats. Everyone climbed out, quickly taking up positions. The landing was sealed off.

Uniformed police gathered around the target door ready to open it. The sergeant knocked on the door. No answer. He knocked again. There was still no answer. He knelt down to the letter box, opening it as he knocked again. "Police! Would you please open the door?" he mouthed through the box. Legal requirements having been met, he nodded to the team as he straightened and moved to the side.

As the door splintered we were up and running, Barry took a step behind me to my right. A yard short of the door I heard Barry laugh and felt a push that propelled me into the sergeant standing against the wall. I just glimpsed Barry getting to the door first. Within the blink of going through the door there was an explosion that threw Barry straight back out. The flat had been rigged. A trip wire had set off a hand grenade. Barry had no chance.

That should not have been Barry. It should have been me. Whatever happened immediately after that I was never quite sure. All that I remembered was vomiting all the way down the stairs, that I was being gripped under both arms and that I was crying like a baby.

The two of us had been together for most of the years since meeting at Hendon Police Training College. We had come back together two years earlier in the Drug Squad. By then Barry had married Sally and was ecstatically happy. My own marriage had come and gone. Although we had been best man at each other's wedding I always felt Sally slightly resented the friendship, so I tried to never intrude into Barry's married life beyond normal involvements.

The funeral was almost two weeks later. I had tried

speaking to Sally but she never responded to my calls. Either her mother, or sister, or someone else answered the phone. I never spoke to her. She never called back. When I arrived for the service I saw that it was a very police affair with full honours. Only then did I realise that despite our friendship I was not closely involved. I wondered why. It hurt.

When it was all over, and all were paying respects to the family, I hung back to have a chance to speak to Sally. As I approached her she looked at me, as if not seeing me, then turned and walked away.

I stood, shocked, mortified and totally at a loss. I felt the tears start to well in my eyes. I heard a voice that I recognised as my own sergeant. From what seemed like the other end of the galaxy it was telling me not to worry. It was just that Sally blamed me. Somehow she knew that it was my turn to go first. It should have been me and Barry should still have been with her.

I went home without going to the wake. Then the pain hit me. Jimsi got me down to Bath, and talked me into a new life.

4

The tall, young man continued walking away from the foyer of Bath Spa Railway Station having turned right. He said his farewells to his companions and continued past more of those queuing for taxis. He walked past the taxis waiting in line for the next passengers. He walked past the length of the station frontage, past the full glass window of the Enquiry Office, and past the end of the building. He turned sharp right towards the archway of the viaduct holding the lines of the station, now immediately above.

Once in the archway he stopped and leaned against the wall. He smiled gently to himself. It had been so easy. No-one had noticed a thing. The two young Japanese girls had been overcome with giggles when he helped carry their bags through the station to the taxi rank. He just left his shoulder bag in amongst their luggage.

Standing six feet two inches in height, blond haired, wide shouldered, slim at the waist, with a slight tan; he looked the picture of a Greek god. He had always loved having that lightly browned tone to his skin ever since his father had worked abroad when he was a young boy. After that it had been regular holidays abroad, usually twice a year. If the tan paled he had taken to the sun parlour, long before it had become fashionable. He was always careful not get too orange looking. He did not appreciate jokes about being tangoed.

Dressed in a soft leather bomber jacket, and fashion faded jeans he looked as if he was just waiting for his girl to arrive. At 23 years old there had been many of them for him. In truth there had been too many for him to remember, or even care about. He could have any woman that he fancied, and he did. He also had more than a few he did not fancy. They had helped fill an empty evening from time to time. He viewed them as expendable amusements. He had no conscience about their use and abuse. After all he never forced any, and they were old enough to make up their own minds.

Life had been good to him. Born of "nouveau rich" parents he had never wanted financially. Born with an intellectual mind he had excelled academically, and gained a Bachelor of Science degree 1 at Bath University. Born healthy and being physically tuned all his life he had shone at sports and now that he had met his parent's requirement of a sound academic degree had carried on to undertake a course in Sports Science at the city's acclaimed sport's university.

Everything had been so good. Now it was so different. A dark glower transformed his features. There would have to be a settlement for what had happened to him. He was not going to endure this alone. Others would have to feel his agony.

The explosion blasted through the air. He felt the air rush by, but with no effect on him. He pushed clear of the wall and headed through the archway, across the car park, over the bridge crossing the canal, and onto the dual carriageway of Claverton Street.

It was such a drag he would have to walk, but there would be no buses passing out of Bath centre in his direction for some time. Normally, from the town, he would have caught the Number 2 bus to Combe Down, then a short walk to the house.

It was a warm Thursday afternoon in May and at 4.20 p.m. he had plenty time to get home for dinner, and the news.

5

Jack Graham bent to tie his shoe lace. It was a nuisance in such a busy situation, but he had to correct it. His whole ethos was concerned with precision.

He had just got off the train from London having been up to Whitehall for a meeting. There was no point returning to his office at the new Ministry of Defence buildings at Abbey Wood, Bristol. It was too late to get back there to just turn round and return home to Bath.

Still, he would not have to be concerned about such considerations for much longer. At 59 years old he only had a few months before entering his sixty first year and retirement. He had enjoyed his career, until the last year, or two. Starting as an apprentice at Devonport Dockyard in Plymouth, when it was a dockyard and not this blasted new terminology of a Naval Base, his forty two years service had seen him progress steadily to become a Senior Ship Construction Engineer. Much of the time he had been based in Bath, his home town, as it had six decades as a Naval Headquarters location arising from the dispersals from London during World War Two.

The essence and satisfaction of the job had remained with him for almost all his career. The design and construction of ships for the Royal Navy had been his boyhood dream. Now the politically motivated privatisation of such work, and the diminishing role to contract supervision had lead to disillusionment. Allied to that the constant demands for performance indicator recording merely exacerbated the distancing from actually being allowed to do the job he had always wanted to do.

He was glad to be getting home at a reasonable time. Later he would go to his main love and recreation at the male choir practice. Tomorrow he hoped to enjoy the opening concert at the Bath Festival.

Unfortunately, Jack was not to see the concert. Nor was he to enjoy retirement. He was not even destined to take one more step from the frontage of Bath Spa Railway Station.

As he started to rise from his stooped position, gently sighing with contentment of his forthcoming plans, he noticed a rather scruffy shoulder bag lying in amongst some very expensive looking luggage beside two Japanese girls. His security training screamed at him that it was all wrong. He had barely registered the thought, nor moved much more than an inch, before six ball bearings blasted through him, snuffing life from him forever.

The time was 4.20 p.m.

6

The two girls chattered excitedly. Their appearance did not necessarily indicate they were not British. After all, the United Kingdom had become such a melting pot of different races that physical attributes no longer defined apparent nationality. So, their very oriental appearance did not signify anything in itself.

However, the chatter was certainly not in English. Equally foreign was much of the writing on their luggage labels. The main clue to their origins was the word "Japan" that did appear on the English section of their labels.

They had been lucky to find their railway carriage had stopped so that as they stepped down they were immediately across from the exit steps. As they had struggled with their baggage a tall handsome man had helped them. He had looked a bit like David Beckham whose picture they both had in their respective bedrooms at home. So handsome, they thought.

Now they stood at the head of the queue waiting for a taxi to take them to their hotel. The trip had been two years in the planning, and now they were following so many of their compatriots who had included Bath in their European tour itinerary.

It was going to be even more special for them as they would go to a number of events over the next few days at the Bath Festival. Both were accomplished violinists and were so looking forward to going to the opening concert the following night.

Both girls lived in Tsuchiura a mid -sized town about ninety minutes north of Tokyo. It is a" new town" lacking traditional appearance but accommodating lots of the features of modern Japan: bars, hostess joints and karaoke bars. Most of the population commuted to work in other cities. So it was with both their fathers. They were of the vast army of workers immaculately suited each morning leaving their homes by six o'clock, not returning until nearer eleven in the evening, after work and compulsory drinks with their bosses and co - workers.

The two fathers were scientists working at nearby Tskuba, Japan's "Science City" home to inventors, scientists, researchers, and the nation's space agency. As such they were well rewarded and sought to give their families all the advantages of modern life. That included sending their children to the best schools, encouraging them in every social, sporting and academic way. Importantly it included the opportunity to travel.

So the two girls arrived in Bath as part of their development, and world wide adventure.

The next taxi in line edged forward. As Kazuko bent over to pick up her bags all the excitement of the holiday died. So did she. Two ball bearings crashed through the top of her head killing her instantly.

Her companion, Yoshimi, was a little luckier, but was left in searing pain, and an injury that would ensure she would not walk freely for a long time to come. A single ball bearing smashed through her right kneecap leaving it in shattered pieces.

The time was 4.20 p.m.

7

The number 2 bus to Combe Down rolled to a stop at the red lights at the bottom of Manvers Street, across from the frontage to Bath Spa Railway Station.

The driver looked at his watch. It showed 4.19 p.m. He hummed to himself. Errol never got stressed about driving his bus through the city. He loved it. He loved his life. He loved his job. He loved everybody. All his passengers loved him.

Errol Grant was not the morose type of bus driver too commonly experienced by the travelling public. He was jolly, helpful, friendly and respected by all.

Errol had a history. It was not one he ever boasted about, but one that somehow everyone on his routes knew.

A second generation West Indian, born in Bristol, he had started to get into trouble as a teenager running with the wrong crowd in St. Pauls. His parents were not happy with him, but he was finding it difficult to break out of the circle he had got himself into. One day he had been kicking his heels around the city and had found himself standing outside the Army recruiting office reading the posters. An alert sergeant had noticed him, came out to speak to him, and got him inside for a chat. By the time Errol walked back out the door he had joined up.

It was a decision he had never regretted for the camaraderie, training, travel, sport and general experience. He had to take plenty abuse from his "friends" initially. That had stopped on one of his early visits home on leave. Someone had pushed too hard only to get the benefit of Errol's training. He never had any bother after that.

His service had included several tours in Northern

Ireland, the Falklands Campaign in 1982, the First Gulf war of 1992, and the Balkans. There were other world wide postings which had been considerably more enjoyable, and safer. Those postings had not added to the impressive row of medals he wore on Remembrance Sunday: the only day he felt it appropriate to get them out. They were not all just campaign medals. He had been recognised for his bravery, but never talked of those days. He always laughed off any conversation heading in that direction by claiming "That was yesterday. You got to live for today, man."

That is what he did, and that was why he loved meeting "his public". Qualified as an HGV and PSV driver before leaving the Army he had taken a job in haulage initially. The money was good but he was away from home too much, and he did not want that any more. He wanted time with his wife and family, so he took to bus driving and found himself back in the West Country, in Bath rather than Bristol.

Things were good. Life at home was good. He had matured from a slim eleven and a half stone to a rounded thirteen stones in just under two years.

As he sat behind the driving wheel waiting for the lights to change he lightly drummed his fingers. Just another hundred yards, or so, and he would be able to spark off all those passengers waiting beyond the station to go up from the city centre to Wellsway, Bear Flat and beyond, towards Foxhill.

He never got that far. Only one ball bearing flew beyond the car parking area at the front of the station. Somehow it traversed between all the people congested there, all the taxis queued up, and all the cars in the pickup zone. Somehow it flew straight across to the number 2 bus and entered the windscreen at an acute angle. Mercilessly it then entered Eroll's very brief remaining life through his temple.

No sniper could have hit him with more fatal accuracy than that random ball bearing.

His wrist watch had just clicked over to show the time as 4.20pm.

8

The pain was unbearable. I wondered if this was what it was like to be crucified. The back of my neck was so stiff, and pain shot up the back of my head. There was no release in trying to move my head, or ease my shoulders. From the base of my neck the pain travelled straight along my shoulders.

Every movement felt as if it was shredding every nerve ending from my shoulders up over my head. I could have cried but knew that would only make things worse. I just wanted it to end, but there was no sign of that happening. It had been with me for more than a day.

The only relief was to take painkillers with lots of water and sleep. I crawled back into bed. It was two in the afternoon. "Please let it finish soon ", I thought, as I covered my head with the bed covers, and tried to sleep.

It took two days for the pain to ease.

9

I felt pressure suddenly being applied to a point low down on the right side of my neck. I heard the gasp from a short intake of breath, just outside my field of vision.

The idle chatter was silenced. There was a flurry of movement that I could hear .The door opened and banged closed. Still the pressure was being applied. Lynda was still there, then.

I knew, instinctively, that something was wrong. Things were not going to script.

I was just a little perturbed. The procedure was being worked on my jugular vein. The old saying of "going for the jugular" and its inference of finality, together with scenes from old action films of unwary sentries having their throats slit flickered across my mind. More amusingly I envisaged myself in a scene from "M*A*S*H" with blood, my blood, spraying the walls.

"Do we have a gusher, then?" I asked.

"Well, no. Not as bad as that, but we've got a little snag. Molly's gone for the doctor. It's nothing to worry about".

Lynda had received me from the ward just a little while before, to insert the Hickman Line. It would save me having dozens of injections, but the offset was the thought of having it inserted through my jugular vein. Lynda was one of a small team responsible for doing that, but with a doctor in close attendance in case of any problems. She had re-assured me it was all routine. It was a regular procedure and she had done over a hundred herself with no problems.

"Please say no more. Don't tempt fate", I said, as I lay on the trolley waiting for her to start. So fate had intervened. Things had gone awry.

"It looks as if I've gone through the wall of the vein. That's why I've got my thumb on your neck, to stop the bleeding. Veins can be quite irregular and I've obviously hit a thin bit. There's no blood on the ceiling, you'll be pleased to know."

The doctor arrived and there was a hushed conference in which I caught the gist of instruction to keep the pressure on for five minutes, then start again. So it was done. The second time there was no problem that did not ease Lynda's embarrassment. It did not ease the mortification she felt, or the pain of no longer being able to say she had done over a hundred procedures without any problems.

She apologised profusely for what had happened. I told her not to worry, it was nothing. It was inevitable it would happen one day. It just seemed equally inevitable it would happen with me.

For the next five months I lived with the Y shaped tube hanging from my chest. I learned to flush it twice a week, injecting the solution into the end caps. Each time I prepared the needle I thought how I could never become a junkie. It was enough for me to inject into piece of plastic. Into my arm? Never!

After my last treatment Peter pulled the tube out. He literally just pulled the tube out. There was a little resistance at first then it just came out. Again pressure was applied for a few minutes to ensure the vein closed over. Thereafter I had a small lump under the skin at the point where tissue had grown like a grommet around the tube.

No matter how else I healed, no matter that my hair grew back, no matter that one day in the future people would look at me and never know what I had gone through, that small lump would always be there as a reminder.

10

The police station in Bath is situated in Manvers Street. Exit the main front doors, cross a small car parking area and you are on the pavement looking straight across the street to a large electrical store. Look left and some one hundred and fifty yards away the railway station stands facing up the street.

From half way down on the other side of the street the bus station dominated the corner, standing in the middle of a one-way traffic system. From the bus stops exiting Railway Street onto Manvers Street traffic can flow turn both ways: right towards the railway station into the one-way flow; left up past the police station in two way traffic.

I found myself out on the pavement, barely conscious of how I got there, but already realising it had not been the wisest use of my limited energy. Traffic was already stopped as far back as where I was standing on my side of the street, but flowing freely on the other side. Uniformed officers streamed past me towards the railway station. Turning my head I saw others running up towards North Parade and Orange Gardens. No doubt they would be ensuring no more traffic came down Pierrepont Street into Manvers Street. I vaguely thought this would be when the contingency plan for city centre disruption would be cranking into gear.

There was a small city bus sitting at the traffic lights at the bottom of the street as it turned ninety degrees into Dorchester Street. The traffic lights were at green and even as I watched there was no move by the bus to get on with its journey.

I walked as far as the next building along before deciding I could not usefully go on. I did not know what I had been thinking. All those months of chemicals pumped into my body to overcome the rogue cells, and I had dashed out as if I was fully fit. I certainly was not.

I looked at the building. It was the Baptist Church. It was surprisingly well known throughout the country, if only by name. There was a time any early morning listener to Radio 2 would have been introduced to the resident reverend on a regular basis by the well known voice of the presenter, Terry Wogan. Such pleasantries did not enter my mind then.

Under the church was a homeless shelter run by Julian House Charity. Each night some thirty to forty unfortunate souls would form a queue to stay in the warmth and comfort until the morning.

I was feeling wretched. I made to sit on the church steps, but realised I should go in the other direction. I got to the edge of the pavement just before I retched up a mouthful of bile. I gulped in air. As I raised myself my eyes crossed with the passenger of the car immediately in front of me. I saw the disgust registered on the woman's matronly face. I saw the unspoken accusation that I had been drinking too much all afternoon. The proximity to the shelter, and my appearance, probably made her think I was one of the dossers. If only she knew, I thought. Not that I was ever too fashion conscious, but I thought I was a bit better dressed than for someone to think I looked that sort of rough. I braced myself and very slowly turned back towards the office.

They did not need me out here. I had no role to play. They might not need me inside either, but I would see. Something nasty had happened. I just knew it. My training, my life, was about being there to help sort out these things. I just had to be able to contribute something no matter how awful I felt.

The thought of that cooling drink taking me one small step back to normality had fled from my consciousness.

11

I slumped across my desk. I felt hot; ashen in temperature, and colour. The desk felt so cool against my forehead. How had it all come to this, I wondered, knowing full well the answer to the question.

It had started so innocuously, so apparently innocently. Just a drying off after a game of squash had been the start. It was not even a serious game; just a bit of exercise and an excuse for a drink with my old friend, Jimsi.

We had been friends for years. We met at Empress State Building in Fulham when I had started working in the MOD. It was all of twenty seven storeys high with the canteen on the twenty sixth. In those days a strong pair of binoculars allowed a bird's eye view into Chelsea Football Club's ground of Stamford Bridge. Unfortunately, at that time, it was hardly worth the bother of trying to get a free viewing.

Both of us came from the same part of the country. Jimsi was born only a few miles further along the coast from Lossiemouth, in Buckie. The personnel department had shown a remarkable, and very occasional, grasp of its function in life and introduced the two of us to each other. Although our time together in the building had not been more than a couple of years we had always stayed in touch. Sometimes we had not seen each other, or spoken, for a year at a time but contact was always warm, and as if the last time had only been the day before. It was Jimsi who, years later, persuaded me to move to Bath to get over that horrendous night at Canary Wharf.

When we had first been introduced Jimsi was named as Jim Gardener. No sooner were we out the door when he said" At hame they ca' me Jimsi.It's family. Ma

27

faither is James, ma gran faither is James. So we're aw cawed different so we ken who we're tauking aboot. Think we're gane tae gate alang fine. Ye can ca' me Jimsi , as weel". So it had been. The only thing of any note about Jimsi that changed over the years was his accent. He refined it and it was difficult, at times, not to think of him a Home counties boy. Only when he was on the 'phone to his family still in the North of Scotland did that lapse, and he reverted to his native Doric.

We had long given up thoughts of playing league squash. It was long since that we had given up the cost and profile of belonging to the Squash club up the hill at Lansdown. Now we were quite happy to book a court at the Sports Pavilion along North Parade, next to the river ,and close by the home to Bath Rugby Football Club. More to the point, it was no more than a quarter mile walk from my office. Jimsi had moved into the world of security within the MOD, and spent too much time in London. That was certainly according to his wife, and substantiated by the declining standard of his play. Plus he had always suffered from asthma, and the additional years were making it harder on him.

Not that I was a goliath of the court any more, either. My police work, fractured time availability, and the repercussions of my many injuries had taken toll on my ability.

So now we just enjoyed the excuse of the sport to sweat a few pints off, then go and replace them at some welcoming hostelry.

The game had gone as so many before. Both of us thrashed around for quarter of an hour with honours even. Then Jimsi had his first gasp of his inhaler and his energy levels started to leave him. There was only one outcome after that, but the never stated etiquette was that it never be more than marginal.

A quick strip off, into the shower, dry off, and then

it started to unravel. It was not the normal quick change and away. I had all but dried myself and was removing my manhood from sticking to my inner thigh. That was such a masculine thing. I had been amused by it for years. The number of men who spent longer than necessary drying and sorting out their hanging bits was unbelievable.

Whether it was them evaluating their current prowess, anticipated prowess, or yearning for what used to be, I had always been amused by the performance. For my own part I had always been a bit self conscious about it and finished as quickly as possible. Equally, I had never been a total practising believer in "man checks" as regularly advised by doctors and medical literature.

That night, as I set myself free, I half thought I felt something different about my testicle. It was almost impossible to think something was wrong on the basis of the fleeting feeling. I stopped. "Ridiculous", I thought, but somehow, something from the depths of my commonsense told me to check.

I, very self-consciously, turned towards the wall gently cupping my hand round my groin. I pulled the skin of the sack tight over my right testicle and felt over the surface with my finger. Nothing unusual was there to be found. It was all very spherical and even .I gently rolled the testicle and checked again. My brow creased. There seemed to be a protrusion. I took my hand away and took a step back as if the tile I had been standing on had just caught fire.

"Don't be so stupid" I said to myself. I gathered myself and repeated the operation on my left testicle. Absolutely uniform in shape it showed no signs of anything unusual. The only thing was it seemed bigger than its partner. I had never thought of the dimensions of testicles. It was not the sort of thing that would occur to me on a day to day basis but I supposed I had always assumed both were much the same size. Certainly no medical examination had ever caused any mention of anything wrong. Certainly no other form of gentle, caressing evaluation, or of aroused demand had ever recoiled.

I moved my hand back to the right and checked again. This time I took more care as I did. It was different!! It was smaller, and on one side was a lump the size of a pea.

I sat down on the bench. As I looked up I saw Jimsi watching me with a questioning expression. I flushed slightly and gulped.

"Jimsi, I think I've a lump on my bollock".

"Well", came the reply in a dry, commanding tone "no point telling me. You better get yourself down to the doctor and get it checked out".

12

Three days after that squash game I had an appointment with the doctor. I felt lucky to have got one in that timescale .It did not do to be too unwell, as the wait for an appointment could be terminal, I had always thought.

Of course, I could not expect everything. The appointment was not with my registered doctor. That would have been too much to be expected. Doctor Hunter was on holiday, again. Perhaps that was the result of being a relatively young, keen practitioner, always at the forefront of new ideas, and a favourite for interviews with the local television stations. Being photogenic and articulate helped. However, the frequent absences were not appreciated that much by his patients.

So I had to wait to see a locum. When my turn came I answered the call and entered a very small consulting room. It was barely big enough to accommodate the desk, with all its attendant computer equipment, two chairs and the couch. I was glad neither I, nor the doctor, had halitosis, or bad body odour. I knew the doctor did not, and no-one had ever told me I had.

"What's the problem?"

"Well, doctor, I'm not sure. It might all be my imagination, and just nothing, but I think I've got a lump on my testicle".

The doctor was already reaching for his rubber gloves. "There's one way to find out. Up on the couch and take your trousers down, then".

Slowly, without wanting to appear too reluctant I complied, pulling my shirt out of the way for good measure. I knew this was the only way to do things, but I still felt self conscious about the process. I felt the doctor's fingers collecting, travelling, weighing and smoothing. First it was to one side, then the other, and back again.

"Okay. Get dressed". After a few moments as I gathered myself together I heard the doctor continue. "Your imagination is not playing tricks. You do have a lump. That is all I can tell you. Given where it is there is every reason to have it fully assessed as quickly as possible. I am going to refer you for a scan at the R.U.H. You should have an appointment within two weeks. If you have not heard within ten days you must, and I repeat must, get in touch with us. Don't worry too much at this stage. This is standard procedure, but we must do things swiftly in case there is a problem, and to ease your mind if there is not". There was no overstatement in the doctor's tone or expression.

I ghosted out of the door and stopped. "Bloody hell", I thought," Just don't panic, yet!"

13

"Now, I can't tell you that we will remove your testicle. That can only be your decision. However, we would recommend it".

A month had gone by since I saw the doctor. Now I was sitting in the office of a consultant oncologist in the Princess Anne wing of Bath Royal United Hospital. There is an old saying that as you get older the policemen look younger and younger. Naturally, I had never subscribed to that view. Now I thought the saying must be more appropriate to medical consultants. The man sitting opposite, advising me to have my testicle removed, looked as if he could hardly be more than twenty three years old, for goodness sake.

The appointment letter for the scan had arrived only four days after seeing the doctor. The date was set for exactly fourteen days after that original visit. Despite myself I was impressed. The appointment time was 10.00 a.m.

To the minute I had been called from the waiting area. Again I had been impressed. It made a mockery of the sniping that was endemic against the National Health Service generally, and against the hospital, in particular, conducted by the local press.

As I entered the room I was conscious of the female staff exiting by another door. I saw the room was in darkness other than the light beamed on the examination bed that awaited me. Somehow, suddenly, strangely it all appeared as a modern torture chamber and I felt a pang of apprehension.

That was misplaced, for the time being, as the radiographer introduced himself very cheerfully. Then came the next request to climb up and, once again, lower my trousers.

"This will be cold. I'm going to place this

jelly on your testicles, and scan over them with this probe. That will relay pictures to this screen which will show us if there is anything to get bothered about".

I saw an instrument in the man's hand that resembled a sophisticated, upturned metal ice-cream cone. Thoughts of women being scanned for babies filtered through my mind.

I gasped as the jelly was applied. It was cold!

I felt the scanner moving. I heard the clickety clack of computer keys as the readings were transmitted to the ghostly grey screen that had come alive just on the edge of my field of vision.

The time passed. One minute. Two minutes. My eyelids drooped. Still the time drifted on until I heard," Finished. Would you like to see what we've got?"

I grunted an assent before manners overruled my initial reaction, and I replied "I think I would".

More clicking of the key pad followed. A handful of tissues was passed to me to clean myself up and get dressed. The process took a little time before I felt I could pull my trousers up, and not leave them embarrassingly stained for public viewing.

"Right, if you look at the screen I'll point out your testicle". Initially the screen was just a fuzz of grey and white flecks, but gradually my eyes started to focus. "Here is your right testicle", as an oval shape was pointed out. I could see that there seemed to be a large white area in the middle of it. I was not mistaken. "That white area in the middle indicates a tumour. I can't say whether it is benign, or malignant. I can only say that it needs to be dealt with. I'm going to recommend you be fast tracked for a consultant's visit".

The young consultant continued outlining how in normal circumstances a small sample would be taken for biopsy and the wound stitched up. "However, with testicles it isn't that easy. It's a major job operating in that area at all. To cut you open then put it all back would not be a great idea if we have to open you up again in a couple of weeks. Neither can we count on an immediate biopsy. The lab boys like to play with their samples, covering all the options. They would like the time to freeze them, pickle them, smoke them and generally play about with them. Not ideal with you lying around with your bits hanging out. It's much better to have it out and do the testing after. Just having one testicle doesn't impair your reproductive ability, if that's a worry to you. We can always insert a prosthetic for you".

The chuckle that started to rise from my throat was cut off in a strangled splutter. At my age I had no ambition to start a family. My brothers had done their bit to ensure the family name would live on, and the family had long resigned themselves to me not sprouting forth on that particular issue.

"No. That's not a problem to me", I said. "In fact, there is no problem in any way. I made the decision it could go a split second after I was told there was a tumour".

The consultant's eyebrows registered his surprise. Obviously he was not used to such clear thinking, nor such objective decision making. "Sure?"

"Absolutely. The options seem pretty limited. Make the effort to live, and maybe walk lopsided, or just take a walk into oblivion. I'm not a chicken any more, but nowhere near ready to call it quits yet. I'll take the chance on being lopsided"

"Give me a minute, and I'll see what I can do", said the young man as he raised himself from his chair and left the room. It took longer than a minute, but before five had elapsed he was back. "That's it fixed for next Friday, nine days time. Okay with you?"

It was, but I had no interest in having a ball bearing replace the lost testicle.

14

The operation had not resulted in me walking lopsidedly. The loss of a testicle was not significant in that regard. However it did leave me moving rather gingerly for a few days. After that it left me moving rather strangely at times as the new hair grew, and the stubble prickled against my pants.

The cut had been made an inch, or so, above my right groin, and was about three inches long. On seeing it for the first time that the dressing was changed I was surprised at how high up it was. Someone had explained to me, sometime through the consultative process, how it would be done, how the testicle would be "pulled" out. I had mentally closed my ears. There was only so much I could take. There was only so much I wanted to take. That detail was just too much information.

I had to take things easy for a couple of weeks. That was the standard advice for an operation in that area. There would be no lifting of any real weight. There would be no strenuous exercise. Nothing was to impair the healing process. That would be the first period of absence from work.

It quickly became one of the more frustrating times I could remember, trying to move more slowly, more carefully. Just two weeks would see me out of the worst of that, and life would get easier. Against that just two weeks would be time enough to get the results of the biopsy.

I did not get the two weeks. On the tenth day after the operation I had a call from Dr.Hunter's secretary. I was requested to call to see the doctor as soon as possible. The next morning I was gently advised I needed to go back to the RUH very soon. The biopsy had shown up the need for more testing. That was to be a bone marrow test.

I was entering a world I had no experience of. Layers were gradually being peeled away, as with an onion. At the kernel was the answer, hopefully. Instinctively I felt that I was being pulled in a way that was far from my choosing. I put such thoughts to the back of my mind. Suspicion was one thing. Conclusions should not be jumped to. I would have to wait for all the evidence to be gathered.

That did not stop me becoming just that little bit apprehensive.

15

There was an increasing level of activity and noise surrounding me. I became aware of it as I slowly recovered from that mad rush into the street.

The logic of the situation came to me. The bomb had gone off literally just down the street. The building I sat in was the city's focal point of law and order. It was bursting into a life that would be unparalleled by any previous experience.

Soon the whole place would be a magnet for people and organisations rarely seen there, and unlikely ever together. There would be an Incident Room beyond any previous imagination. The nature of the crime would mean the involvement of groups way outside any normal activity. Scotland Yard's Anti-Terrorist team would be there, too. Communications links would have to be priority cleared to London's Incident Rooms involving MI5 and other Security Services. They would run investigative teams beyond the immediate Bath activity as well as wider intelligence probing.

On the ground there would be local "house to house" enquiries. Not that there were many residences in the immediate area: more shops and businesses. There would be a swarm of police out on the streets. Reinforcements would be arriving from every corner of the Avon and Somerset force, and beyond.

Now I was sitting like a wet paper bag when I should be involved. They had probably forgotten I was still around; just unconsciously overlooked that I was back at work. This was a situation I had background and experience to contribute. I could not just be left on the sidelines.

I lurched to my feet feeling a moment of giddiness. Uncertainly I navigated around the furniture and headed up the corridor. The door to the Detective Inspector's office was wide open letting me see four bodies standing over the desk, already pouring over piles of papers.

The sharpness of my knock on the door surprised even me, and those in the room. Four pairs of eyes swung towards me registering surprise, then shocked concern. I saw it, but could not understand why they should look at me like that. It must just be the bomb had unnerved them all.

"Boss, what can I do to help?" I asked, as I gently swayed against the door. Ian Welsh glanced around the table, seeing the same concern in the other's eyes as he also projected. He stepped away from the table and moved towards the door.

"You okay? You look awful". Glancing back at his colleagues he excused himself for a minute. "Let's go down to your office".

When we got there we sat down. Welsh sat down. I just collapsed into the chair.

"I'm fine" I replied indignantly, knowing within it was a lie. "I just want to do my bit. I'm okay to help".

"Maybe you do, but not today. You're washed out. You're going home. I don't want you on my conscience. There are plenty others. Just because this has gone off doesn't change your situation. You are just back after all you've been through".

"Go home! Get your rest. If you feel up to it come in tomorrow. We'll see how things shape tonight. Maybe something will come up you can help with. If you're not up to it stay at home. Understand?"

The apparent rejection hit me hard. Here I was offering to do what I was supposed to do, and being turned away. It was like the time I turned up for treatment and I was turned away because my blood counts were not strong enough. I was judged not strong enough to cope. Then I had been shocked that my body had been found wanting. The trouble was this time I really knew it to be true.

Anyway, Ian Welsh was not a good man to argue with. Not that he was an overly big man, though well built, but because of his previous career. Before joining the police he had served in the Army. To be specific he had finished his time with a spell in the S.A.S. If anyone in the station knew about death, and how to administer it, Ian did.

"Okay, I'll go". As I said it I wondered how I would manage. I could not walk up steep Lansdown Hill. There would be chaos trying to get on a bus, if any were around. I doubted if there was much chance of a taxi. There would be no chance of a casual lift in a patrol car. I sighed as I reached into my pocket for my mobile to 'phone Jimsi.

Chance was a fine thing. Jimsi was in London on a Security Conference. Niki said she would come to collect me at the corner of North Parade. I just managed the hundred yard walk.

16

Niki nagged at me all the way home. I looked terrible. I did not look fit to be left alone. I should come back with her and have something to eat. I could just grab some fresh clothes and stay the night with her and James. As a southern girl she had never quite accepted his family name. In truth by the time they met Jimsi had realised to get on he had to become more of an Anglophobe, and had taken to using his baptismal name.

I appreciated the concern but I just wanted to be alone. I did not want the company, really. I did not want to have to think about anything beyond what was pounding through my head. I was annoyed. I was annoyed at being sent home. I was annoyed that I knew my condition was such that I had to be sent home.

Niki dropped me off with a final admonishment that I should get some rest, and take care of myself.

I needed something to eat but had no energy to cook. I compromised with a meal of some beans on toast. By the time I sat down I just caught the highlights at the end of the News at 6.30.

So I just sat, totally exhausted, in the chair I had fallen into that first time I got home from chemotherapy treatment.

17

The glass of whisky sat on the coffee table. At the far end of the table. It was not just any whisky, but a malt, and a good malt, at that: The Glenlivet, 12 year old. It was argued by many as one of "the" whiskies. A Christmas present from my father it had been drunk from sparingly, marking special occasions. It was a Speyside, naturally.

I had tried the offerings of all the regions, from the heavy, iodine taste of the Western Isles to the mild tones of the Lowlands but he had become a Speyside man. It was not just because of my birthplace, but I just preferred the clean taste and colouring.

I was home after my first course of chemotherapy. It had been an overnight stay so the team could monitor my initial reaction to the various drugs. It had gone very well. No violent sickness. In fact, I had no sickness at all. No adverse reaction to anything. I felt pleased and relieved in equal measure.

There had even been a bit of fun when I had gone in for my first session. Someone else was already in the suite hooked to a drip. Casual conversation soon determined the man was on his sixth month of treatment. The noticeable thing about him was that he had such a good head of hair.

As Ally, the nurse, connected my line I said to her "Thought you folks said I would lose my hair? Look at him. Six months treatment and look at his hair". Ally looked me straight in the eye. She tapped my knee as an old school mistress would chastise an errant pupil. "You will", she said. The certainty in her voice did not invite any argument.

Now I was home. Jimsi had collected me, again inviting me to stop over at their place, but I felt that would be too soon. There may be a day that I would be glad to accept. Not just yet, though.

So after settling back in I thought I would have a wee dram. It wasn't a celebration, but more of a "well done, so far". That seemed fair. I poured the whisky, loving the glugging sound as it came out of the bottle. I added the slightest drop of water to release the flavour, before sitting down by the coffee table.

I raised the glass to within an inch of my mouth and the attraction died.

It was as if I had been slapped. The aroma from the glass was not the warm, beckoning amber I so enjoyed. It was a gut wrenching stench that made me want to heave. I placed the glass down and pushed it to the far end of the table. I eyed it as if it was a cobra waiting to strike at me. I was suspicious, frightened to move. I could not believe it was like this, but it was. The thought was dawning that perhaps things were not so well.

Little did I realise how much things would get worse. It would be many a long month before my love affair with whisky was rekindled.

18

As I poured the whisky away, and that added to my anguish, I came to accept the past few days had been a phoney war. In fact, every stage had seemed so innocuous in itself that I had been completely unaware of how big a black hole I was being sucked into. It was a world way beyond my comprehension, awareness, or feeling. Yet, around me those past few days had been the reality of what I was now involved in. My ignorance had stopped me appreciating that what I saw could equally apply to me.

The stories, and condition, of those in the ward had still been beyond me. I lay in a bed surrounded by men battling cancer, but that was them. It wasn't me! I wasn't like them. They really had it. I just had a little bit of a problem that wasn't really that bad. I hadn't even felt ill, after all. They were all struggling. I was as fit as an ox. I was sure of that, in my own mind. It was never going to affect me the way it did them.

As I stood at the sink the face of Willie Henderson came into my mind. Poor old Willie! I felt so badly about making Willie cry.

Willie must have been well into his seventies. The first thing that struck me about Willie was the back of his hands and arms. They were mottled black and purple with bruising. I had seen that effect on many a junkie, but never the whole arm, like Willie. Not only must the continued injections have caused the old man so much discomfort but he had been fitted with a catheter. It did not fit well with him, causing him real pain. Willie was in trouble.

He was old, and weak. He needed rest to keep

up some strength for the fight. The trouble was his family wanted to look after him and keep him company. They came in waves .The first landing of the day was sharp at 8 a.m. Then they came in synchronised shifts over the next twelve hours. At times Willie could do no other than eventually fall asleep with exhaustion. They were helping kill him with their affection.

Willie had a pronounced accent. It did not belong to Bath, but there was no doubting his family were all locally raised. When I had a chance to talk to Willie it turned out the old man had come south forty years ago for work as an engineer in the coal mines still operating in Somerset at the time. It was the old story. He met a local girl, married and stayed. The pits closed but other work had always been there to be had.

The thing was Willie was a Fifer born and bred. Our chat touched on the history of the old Kingdom, the ancient capital of Dunfermline, Kinghorn, Falkland and its royal palace, and St. Andrews. As we talked of the old towns and the old ways Willie was overcome .Tears seeped from the corners of his eyes. Emotion was proving too much for the old man, so I thought it best to excuse myself with a need to go to the bathroom.

When I got back Willie had fallen asleep. The conversation had never been resumed.

Directly across from me in the mini-ward of four beds was Cyril Smythe. It was pointed out quite emphatically it was not Smith. Cyril was a large, loud man who liked the sound of his own voice. He was going to sue the world. He was going to sue the nurses for not looking after him quickly enough, or well enough. Other people needing attention were of no interest. He was going to sue the hospital for anything and everything. He was going to sue the pharmaceutical companies for selling drugs that did not provide an instant cure for his condition.

Cyril was an angry man who did not take kindly to his diagnosis, nor to his situation. He was not happy with his lot, but rather than work at overcoming it was lashing out those trying most to help him. After the initial introductory chat I did my best not to get into conversation with Cyril.

In the bed to my left was a man I never got to know. Most of the time the bed was curtained off. When it was not the man was invariably unconscious. I never got to know the man's name.

As I stood at the sink I was not to know I would never see any of those men again. During my treatments over the coming months I noticed many little groups who greeted each other warmly and who had obviously shared experiences that bonded them. That clearly did not apply to everyone. When I saw those groups I would often think of Willie, particularly. Whether it was just mistiming of appointments, or ill fortune that we never met again was something I always chose to leave unasked.

19

He was half way up Ralph Allen Drive, and he was struggling. The jacket had long since been taken off. His T-shirt was showing distinct signs of dampness under the arms and down the centre of his back. His forehead was beaded with sweat and his hair turning into rat's tails at the back of his neck, as it got damper.

His steps were becoming shorter and he found he was swaying from side to side as he stepped forward. Another half mile of steep incline to the top of the hill had to be endured. It was damnable to feel like this.

He remembered virtually dancing all the way up just a few weeks previously. He started to feel giddy and to his great shame accepted he would have to rest. He sat on the wall and let his head drop, slowly, methodically drawing in large gulps of fresh air. He was not so far out of condition to forget the basics of proper breathing.

It did. By the time he stumbled to the top of the hill, turned left, then right and walked another two hundred yards to the house he was exhausted. The shirt was sticking to his back. His hair was plastered to his head. His Adonis good looks had forsaken him. The slight tan had been overtaken by a greyish palor.

He staggered in through the front door and called a greeting. There was no reply, for which he was grateful. He did not want either of his parents to see him as he was. Just in case, though, he had his story long since prepared.

At the bottom of the stairs he swayed gently. Upstairs for a shower and freshen up first, or to the drawing room to get the television news, he wondered. He could not be bothered going all the way to the back of the house to switch on the kitchen television. There did seem time to catch the news. He slowly dragged himself across the drawing room and fell into the sofa. The remote control was, uncharacteristically, lying there and the machine on standby. "The old man must have been having a quick look this morning "he thought. His mother would never have been so tardy.

The screen flickered on and he pushed the button for BBC News 24. He heard the news before he saw it. "......killed and twenty seriously injured. The injured are being taken to hospitals in Bath and Bristol. Some have injuries which are likely to result in major surgery, and possible amputation".

Just then the answer flashed across the screen as a headline describing how a device had exploded at Bath Spa Railway Station at 4.20 p.m. that afternoon killing three people and injuring many more.

He smiled wanly. Three was not great, but as a practice run it was not too bad. Now it was time for a shower, change, and get himself together before the old ones got home. He would have to play the dutiful son for a few hours tonight before going to bed early.

Maybe they could have a bottle of champagne as a little family celebration. He had lots planned for the morrow, and another empty champagne bottle could be useful.

20

The Six O'clock News was just starting as he slipped onto the settee. He was still alone in the house but a shower and change of clothes had made him feel more human again.

Almost distractedly he heard the newsreader say that" a device had exploded at Bath Railway Station". That was overlaid by a brief picture of the scene; police cars blocking the road, a bus just beyond them, some taxis sitting at the station entrance, a large white van in the parking area, figures in white over suits searching the ground.

Other news headlines passed over his head as he settled more comfortably, waiting for more detail. Disappointingly there seemed to be no more news than he heard before. Three killed. Over twenty seriously injured. There had been no claims of responsibility. That seemed to be a source of confusion to the news team and the authorities.

The front door rattled as someone entered. His mother walked into the room. She came over behind him laying her hand on his head very briefly. They had always had a distant sort of relationship, and that had become more pronounced over the past few weeks, so it was no surprise to him that the cuffs of her £300 "working suit" should brush so fleetingly against his hair. She would still be losing herself in whatever image she was working on in her capacity as a senior executive in the glossy magazine trade.

"How are you today, darling? Isn't it awful? A bomb going off in Bath!"

She was already halfway back towards the door without waiting for a reply." Would you like a drink? I'm going to have one".

His face had remained impassive throughout. Now it twitched around the corners of his mouth.

"Yeah", he called back. "How about a champagne?"

21

COBRA had met briefly at 8.30 p.m. The Home Secretary sat at the head if the table. Despite the name being derived from "Cabinet Office Briefing Room A" the meeting was held in a meeting room of the MOD Building.

Although the group's responsibility was described as a civil contingencies committee the siting of the bomb in a MOD Headquarters location, and previous terrorist attacks on armed forces bases had lead to the decision to meet where it had. Political nicety was maintained by keeping the chairmanship in strictly non military orientated spheres until things were better defined.

From the Home Secretary down each side of the table were ministers, senior police officers from both civil and military bodies, Intelligence chiefs and secretariat staff. The meeting was short. It amounted to a resume of what had happened, the lack of any intelligence on pre-warning, the lack of intelligence on any suspects, the setting up of London based Incident Rooms to cast a wide net on intelligence gathering, and to link with the local crime scene.

The Public Relations team were directed to be discreet with the release to the media.

Little did any of them know they were involved with a new special agent playing by his own rules and his own game. His position in the game was by self appointment, and he was representing deluded self justification.

22

It was ten o'clock. The national news was being presented on television.

"Earlier this evening a special meeting of the government's emergency committee, COBRA, was held under the chairmanship of the Home Secretary. It was called as a consequence of the bomb which exploded at Bath Spa Railway Station late this afternoon in which three people were killed. There have been no reported claims of responsibility from any organisation. Indeed, it is a mystery why the bomb should have been targeted in the Georgian city at all.

The meeting was held at the Ministry of Defence Building in Whitehall and here to tell us more is our reporter Simon Witherspoon."

A picture of a man holding a microphone came on the screen. Behind him was a set of steps leading to large glass doors guarded by armed police officers. His report re-iterated what had been regularly reported across the media for the previous five hours, re-affirmed everything that the main news presenter had said, but failed to provide anything further. The reason for the bomb was a mystery. It followed no previous experience. The person, or persons, or group responsible were unknown. It was unusual for no claim of responsibility to be lodged. That seemed to indicate it was not the work of activists of any known group, or interest.

So the feature went on adding nothing of value, but providing plenty of conjecture and scope for more fertile imagination to fill columns of newsprint in the following day's newspapers.

The individual responsible was not looking for recognition. At least he was not then. Nor was he in a position to hear it. He had already gone to bed. The effort of getting up the hill had taken its toll, and he needed to be fresh for the morrow. He had much more to do.

Downstairs his parents sipped the last of their wine and agreed it was damnable that such a thing could happen in Bath. In fact, it was so bad his father was very strongly inclined to write to "The Times" about the state of anarchy overtaking the country. He declared he would write similarly to the local press, before flicking over the channels to see if there was anything more entertaining elsewhere.

Across the other side of the city someone else was feeling the effects of the day. I had also heard that COBRA had been convened. I had dozed off earlier but the introduction to the News had woken me. I looked at the TV screen across the same coffee table where the whisky had been placed. I remembered my thoughts of the cobra that day. COBRA. What a coincidence.

Just then all I needed to do, all I wanted to do, was get to bed and sleep.

23

"Gas, gas, gas"

The cry echoed up and down the line of trenches. The soldiers quickly laid down their mess tins and cups before reaching for their gas masks. There was no distinction in the levels of apprehension between the veterans, who had survived earlier attacks, and the newly arrived replacements, who had only heard about it before arriving at the hell of the Western Front 1916.

The duck boards allowed the sticky mud they lay on to ooze over the sides. The banks of the trenches were constantly eroded by trickles of soil adding to that mud. Everything was dank and wet. All that held any semblance of normal life was the relative brightness of the sky. Now that was to be eclipsed by the suffocating, murderous infiltration of mustard gas.

The smoke turned to cloth as I pulled the white blanket up to his chin. I had awoken from my sleep as the cloud of gas was beginning to roll over me.

"The trouble with this treatment is it allows too much time to read and sleep", I thought. I was halfway through my second full week's treatment of methotroxate. That day I had come across a newspaper article describing how chemotherapy had been born out of the horrors of the battlefield.

More than twenty years after the end of World War 1 post mortem studies on soldiers exposed to mustard gas found that their lymph systems had been greatly suppressed. Experiments, based on that finding, had shown that some poisons could overcome lymph cancers. The final evidence was when a patient had been injected the tumour he was suffering from just shrank away. The creation of Chemotherapy had begun.

In the early days the approach lacked sophistication. The treatment was oblivious to what it did. Healthy cells were killed as energetically as the bad. The side effects were traumatic, but better than the only other option of dying.

I had already declared against accepting that option, and although research had refined the drugs used the effects could still be exceedingly unpleasant .Of that I had become too well aware.

24

Half past two in the morning. The ward was in darkness except for my light. Another bad night trying to get sleep. That was no surprise given that there was no real difference between day and night. There was no work time, no rest time. Life revolved around treatment times,twenty four hours a day. I was permanently attached to a drip, always having to take my "friend" Stephen whenever I went to the toilet, to wash, or do anything away from the bed.

Stephen and I were inseparable. I had named the drip stand in recognition of the book "The Stand", by Stephen King. It amused me in a macabre sort of way, which was quite fitting. I enjoyed the author's work and the darkness of his circumstances made for a relationship.

That was not my choice of reading that night. That night it was someone much closer to home. I had been slow to discover the books of Ian Rankin on the cases of Detective Inspector Rebus. In truth I had stayed away from them long enough because the more I was cajoled to read them the more I rejected the idea. Sheer bloody mindedness, really. Or "thrawn" as they would have said back home.

Rebus' operating base around Edinburgh was only marginally familiar to me. The geography of the city centre I could visualise, but further out was lost territory to me. What I could always follow was the detective's excursions back to his home in Fife. The names of the towns rolled off: Kelty, Lochgelly, Lochore, Crossgates, Strathmiglo,Milton of Balgonie, Thornton, Dysart and, of course, Rosyth, home of the now departed Royal Naval Dockyard whose time really came and went in less than a century from the early 1900's.

All those places brought back memories, particularly of my mid teens playing for glory in the Kirkcaldy and District Amateur Football League. Those were the days of fun and freedom! Not all the venues had been as pleasant as those of St. Salvatores at St. Andrews University. Some had been pretty rough in those days. More than a few of the players were of the same ilk.

I closed the book. The print was blurring and I could not get it into focus. The print was not blurring at all. It was my eyes at fault. It was just another consequence of the chemotherapy I had been warned about.

Whilst Old Chemo could dictate my physical well being it could not master my mind. At times like this I found my imagination going into overdrive. It soared and dipped branching off in new directions almost at a whim; sometimes doubling back, other times just taking another tangent.

I had read a book of short stories featuring Rebus. There was one about an old army officer who had his car blown up. The plot was based on the assumption that the IRA had tracked him down. Not so. It turned out the old boy had contrived the explosion himself. No matter about that. The point was I remembered there was a line about where there were terrorists there would be bombs, because there would be targets.

Cancer was a bomb to many people. So was there a targeting process? Was there somewhere a space age office like that of an arch criminal featured in something like a James Bond film, with a Controller of the Big C zooming his satellite cameras down on various cities, towns, villages, and farms?

"Ah, nice looking girl. Let's shoot her a bit of breast cancer. That'll show her".

"Look at him! Fancies himself a bit. Prostate for you, my boy!"

"Now, that's a nice smoky bar. Eeny meeny, every second one with a cigarette, lung cancer. Scientists think they know about that so that'll keep them going. Young barman not smoking? No cigarettes in his pocket. Non-smoker, in fact. Give him a shot anyway. That'll give them something to think about"

My imagination touched down on terra firma. "Not likely" I thought, but with a lingering doubt about the absurdity of it. After all there had been no sensible answer as to how it had got to me.

All they could tell me was it could have been anything from a knock to a cold. It was the $64000 question. Where did it come from? Now I was another adding to the statistic that one person in three was walking around with cancer: whether they knew it, or not.

25

The morning broke to clear skies with a promise of another fine day.

He rolled across the bed. He picked up his watch from the bedside table: 6.04. That was good for him. He needed time. He needed to get some work done in the garage early, make an appearance for a lecture, get back for a sleep, and then it would be party time. Only this time the party would be different. It was to be a one off. Never to be repeated, a headline grabber, if ever there was one. Oh yes, he would make his mark tonight. This would be a night of conquests beyond any he had experienced before, and so, so different.

He needed to be alert for what he had to do. He went down to the shower room. The water had to be just right. Not warm enough to make him feel too relaxed afterwards, not so cold to shock him. It had to be just so. As he dried himself off he saw again the subtle change in his body. The physique was slowly disintegrating. Many would have been pleased to look as he did then, but he knew he was losing it. His teeth clenched as he gently felt the small scar low on his back before he wrapped the towel round his waist.

In the bedroom he chose clean jeans and T shirt. Both sets of yesterday's clothes were in the laundry basket. It may be helped make a lot of ironing but that was what the help got paid for. These would join them before the end of the day, in the same sweat sodden condition.

He heard his parents moving about their en-suite bedroom. They would be leaving soon. His father had to overcome the inconvenience of the railway station being closed. Normally on a Friday he took the small car to the station to catch the train up to London for the weekly board meeting. Today he would probably have to drive out to Chippenham, or go back to Bristol. There would be no way he would be getting on the emergency bus service. Such a drag for him. He would be away soon, that much earlier than normal.

His mother would take the other town car and park in the NCP car park on Corn Street. That was her chosen spot normally, but there would be more competition for spaces. The multi- storey car park behind the bus station, only some 300 yards away, was likely to still be sectioned off. Anyway she would leave at the same time as his father. She always did, always would, even if it was 3.30 in the morning. Necessity had long given way to habit.

He decided to wait until they had left. He lay back on the bed looking at the ceiling, going over the preparations in his mind. The ingredients of the mix had been easy to obtain. He had borrowed the car for a drive the previous Saturday. He knew exactly where to go. Farm shops around the area had been visited. Mole Valley Farmers at Standerwick had been particularly fruitful. He had been careful to only buy quantities that would not excite any interest, or remembrance, of the purchase. Then it was on to those old fashioned ironmongers in Warminster and Devizes. He resisted the temptation to buy ball bearings, and other shrapnel, at those places. There was a chance someone would remember the combination. He had ball bearings in the garage but not enough. He had decided to make do with nuts and bolts. It would still have the same effect. It would be a bit like grapeshot from the old cannons. So he had returned to Bath and obtained all the necessary bits at Homebase.

There were enough champagne bottles. He had recovered sufficient from the re-cycling bin for what he wanted. Last night's had just completed the set of six, thank you very much. He was not sure he could carry more than that. He doubted if the picnic hamper could safely carry more than that either.

The timing mechanism had been a challenge, but he got by. He had wandered the town during the week calling into all the little shops in the back streets and arcades gradually buying what he wanted; slim watches that would slip through the neck of a champagne bottle.

The most important ingredient he did not need to buy. It was all in his head. The knowledge of how to make his cocktail go with a bang had been provided through his education. His degree would not be entirely wasted: at least, not to his mind.

26

The front door opened. There was a muttered conversation as people exited. There was no shouted goodbye. There had been no call to his room to see him before leaving for work. He had not expected there would be. They would have expected him to sleep through until it suited him to get up for his lecture.

Now the coast was clear he raised himself, gathered the watches from his dresser drawer and headed for the kitchen. On the way he called into his parent's room for a handful of his mother's make up removal cotton wipes. He found a cover and spread it over the table. It would be easier to wipe clean when he had finished. He recovered the empty champagne bottles from where he had carefully stashed them behind the full ones. He opened the table drawer and took out the corks saved from those very bottles. He matched the watches to the bottles. Lastly he took the kitchen scales, small funnel and scoop, laying them strategically around his intended working area.

Satisfied that all was in order he left by the back door for the garage. There he gathered up his purchases and carried them back to the kitchen. It surprised him that it took three trips. By the time he had finished there was a fine dew already forming on his brow. He wiped it away with his forefinger. There was a degree of exasperation in that, and he knew he had to control it. He should have been able to do all that so easily. Now it had become an effort.

He placed all the ingredients in the order he would need them. He decided he would do a production line. Each ingredient mixed and filled to each bottle as it was needed. The final action would be sealing each bottle with a cork.

He took pleasure in knowing how to do what he was intent on. He was amused by the poor saps that had to research the internet to learn how to make a basic bomb. Equally he was bemused by those who had to go all the way to Pakistan, or Afghanistan, to be taught by some zealot on the simple chemistry of what to do.

The best bit, of course, was saved for those who did all that then made a mess of the whole operation. That was truly pathetic. That was not going to happen to him. Last night had been a trial run. It had worked. Admittedly there would be a slight change today. He needed the watches to set things for a specific time. Last night he had set a short fuse in his shoulder bag.

Meeting those Japanese girls had been a bonus, making it so much easier to drop it off unnoticed.

He started the production. First to go in was the shrapnel, wadded in with the cotton pads pushed in by the end of a wooden spatula. Then the mixing began. On the News it would be described as a "fertilizer bomb". They could call it what they liked. He was not the least concerned. What did bother him was the effort. The concentration and tension was making him sweat. He noticed his hands were trembling. That had to be a sign of why he was doing this. Again the thought went through his mind that it was not fair. There had to be a balancing.

He stopped and breathed deeply. Sweat dripped from his nose. More stung his eyes. He wiped it away and rose from the chair. He stretched and unconsciously his right hand fell to that small wound on his back. Maybe he should have had the mole removed a lot sooner. This was no good. He needed a sweat band. Having sorted himself out he returned to the chair. Not much more to do, he thought. Just finish this for now and get along to the Uni.

When he finished, and cleaned up, only the filled

bottles, watches, and corks were left on the table. It was only 9.30. It was too early to set the watches. He would do that later. In the meantime he put everything away just in case someone came back, or his mother had asked the help to come in for some reason.

He went back upstairs, washed, put on another T shirt and deposited another in the laundry basket.

27

COBRA reconvened at 08.30 precisely. Some members had been to bed for an almost normal length of sleep. Others had to make do with considerably less.

Sir Alan Brown, Metropolitan Police Commissioner and thereby Head of Anti-Terrorism in the country had the least amount as he fretted over the lack of intelligence on the case. The lack of fore warning coupled to the lack of any claim of responsibility for the outrage was unnerving.

He had very little progress to report and what he did have was puzzling. When called upon to report he openly confessed the lack of background knowledge in all the associated bodies responsible with gathering such information. Nor did he feel comfortable with imparting what little information had been passed to him in the hour before the meeting.

"The only thing I can tell you is that from the scene of crime reports it is clear the device was intended to kill and maim in the most horrific way. A number of ball bearings have been recovered from the scene. They match those that have been removed from the injured. It seems the device was intended as a shrapnel shot.

Also found have been shards of green glass. It seems that bottles, possibly wine, or even champagne bottles, were used to contain the explosives.

The concern has to be that this attack was carried out by an individual with a personal agenda. If that is so we are looking for the proverbial needle in a haystack."

The meeting concluded with many concerned looking faces exiting the room. The public relations communiqué was extremely short, giving those looking for news very little to report, but plenty scope to speculate.

28

"Good morning, good morning, good morning. Come in and take a seat." The voice was warm and cheerful, with a slight accent. It was hard to be precise but it sounded as if the speaker was from Eastern Europe.

The voice came from a man sitting at the desk Harry usually used. He was round faced, with red cheeks, tight curled grey hair which was thinning considerably, gold rimmed glasses perched precariously on the end of his nose, allowing full view of humorous, twinkling eyes.

"I am pleased to meet you, at last. I am Doctor Knightley"

So this was the man, the main consultant. To date all my treatment had been transmitted by Harry, who had always made it clear that everything was guided by Dr. Knightley. Now I was in the presence of the man who was masterminding my fight with cancer. I wondered if that meant I was in for some significant news.

I sat down and looked at the face that was smiling back at me. "I suppose you must have been wondering why you are having such unusual treatment".

My eyebrows shot up in surprise. I had not realised that there was anything unusual about my treatment. I had been into the day centre and the ward enough to notice that treatment was far from uniform. Some came in for a few minutes, others for the day. Not all were using the same drugs. Still that did not give me any reason to think my treatment was unusual.

I had fleeting thoughts that cancer was like divorce. People used the words in a generic sense, but as I had learned divorces could be amicable or vicious. The factors and personalities meant no two divorces were identical. So it was with cancer. Every case was individual depending upon what was under attack, the physical state of the patient, the age of the individual, and the time taken to identify the illness. From somewhere I had learned there were over 200 different types of cancer which could attack some 60 different parts of the body.

I noticed that there was a third person sitting in the room. A lady was sitting behind the door. A small smile pulled at her lips seeing my surprise. I felt the humour of the situation. I realized that she knew what I was thinking, and that was by me knowing that I knew that she knew.

"Er, no, I didn't"

"Oh, yes. I've only had three cases of your kind in the past five years and now I've got two of you together."

That confused me. I had not considered testicular cancer to be that unusual. I knew of many cases reported in the newspapers, even of professional sportsmen who had recovered to resume their careers.

"Yes, testicular lymphoma is not very common. In fact it is quite a rare form of extramodal lymphoma. If it should return it could be very serious. That is why we are giving you such strong measures."

As I left the office the lady came out behind me. "That surprised you, didn't it? By the way I'm Linda. I'm with McMillan Nurses."

That was my second surprise of the day. I had always associated McMillan with palliative care for the terminally ill. Surely I was not headed in that direction.

"Don't worry! I'm not here for you. I'm sitting in on all Dr. Knightley's appointments this morning for case studies. He probably forgot I was there."

"You gave me a wee turn there, I confess. Can you tell me something? I noticed Dr. Knightley seemed to have a foreign accent that doesn't quite match with his name".

Linda gave a throaty chuckle.

"Don't you know the story? It's very romantic. You're right. He's actually Polish, but he uses his wife's proper name. She's an actress. She was in Poland making a film when they met. Although he was a doctor even then he was also a bit of an amateur thespian. He got a small part in the film, probably because he could speak English. According to Joan, that's his wife, he followed her around for ages before he got up the courage to speak to her. She was beginning to think he was in the Secret Police detailed to watch her. Anyway, once they got talking it was pure romance. They married and he moved over here, but it wasn't quite as easy as that, of course. He still does a bit of acting, but strictly amateur productions, never in here".

I saw Linda often in passing during the months. I was just glad I never had to have a meaningful conversation with her about my situation.

29

I was back in the room with Harry. It was my first pre treatment consultation. I had already had my blood tested. My height and weight had been checked. It was a routine that I would get used to. Every time I went in for a consultation I would go through the same routine.

Harry was by himself. This was the start of the real business. The advisory counselling was over. Now it was about joining the mainstream of cancer care. I had recognised it as I sat in the waiting room seeing so many joining me. So many looking ill, so many displaying so many different attitudes. I had picked out the worriers while admiring the warriors. I had been especially taken by the women who had forsaken a wig and wore their bandanas as if they were a band of bravadoes.

Already I had sensed that to be a cancer sufferer gave entry to a mutual support club. I was buoyed by the feeling.

Without knowing he was doing it Harry had attacked that state of mind. First he had brought out all the necessary papers for consent to the treatment.

"You will be getting lots of intravenous treatment. If we tried to give you an injection every time your veins would become extremely bruised and sensitive. We propose to fit you with a Hickman Line. That goes straight into a vein in your neck and is inserted deeply enough to keep it safe. Effectively it is a long tube that splits into a Y to allow us two feeds into you at any one time. That will make it easier to administer the chemotherapy around the clock. You will need to flush it to keep it clean, but we will show you how to do that".

"So, you are almost ready to start. You'll just need

to hand this prescription into the pharmacy to get your tablets. Anything else you want to know?"

There was. Over the past few days I had noticed a number of little lumps , almost like blisters, but firmer, coming up on my right leg. I showed them to Harry.

"Don't worry about them. The therapy will clear them in a few days. I see you also have a little psoriasis on your knee. That will go as well",

"Can't be all bad then", I thought to myself.

30

I woke, but my eyes stayed shut. I tried to open my eyelids but there was no real response. I felt them flicker a couple of times before the mechanisms closed down.

My head slumped further back in the pillow. Slowly I did a roll call of my body parts.

Eyelids were heavy and refusing to open.

Shoulders were stiff, sore and refusing to move.

Elbows were screaming with pain.

Back was aching.

Kidneys were claiming to have been kicked black and blue.

Hip bones were taking sympathy action with elbows.

Knees and ankles seemed to feel it obligatory to join forces with his elbows. The joints were a union unto themselves.

To finish it all off my right calf was twitching, threatening to go into cramp.

I was relieved that my left calf was still on my side, scant consolation that there was in that. I rolled back. It was so much better not to move.

That was no good to me. My brain, my conscience and my training were all telling me I had to move. I had things to do. I had to get to work. I had to help. No cancer fallout was going to stop me doing my job. They had said I had beaten the cancer, so there was no way I could lie in that bed just because my body was suffering from yesterday's exertions.

I gathered what strength I had and rolled out of the bed. The shock of hitting the floor jerked my body alive and my eyelids shot open. Then they closed. My head rolled to the side to rest against the mattress. I groaned. Good intentions started to desert me, but duty stopped the unrest, reinforcing the resolution I needed.

It took an hour before I was ready. "Don't think I'll be available for selection this weekend", I thought, oblivious to the fact the season was over. It gave me a sense of ironic humour all the same. My brain had slowly worked out there was no way I could walk to work. Neither did I have any inclination to stand waiting for a bus, if any were going all the way I needed.

I reached for the 'phone and called my preferred taxi firm. My favourite operator answered. There was no need for introductions. My voice was enough for recognition. "Morning, Molly. Any chance of a taxi, to as near as you can get me to work?"

By 9.30 I was in the office, surrounded by bedlam.

31

It was my first night in for the Methotroxate treatment. Eventually, it had come around.

I had arrived four days earlier, later in the day than expected. The advised early morning call to confirm bed availability had received a negative response. There was no room for me, but I had to call back at 11 o'clock. Then the news was more encouraging. I had to come in after lunch. I duly reported in and was shown to a side room of my own. My blood was taken for testing. Just after that my world crashed over my head.

My blood count was not strong enough to allow the start of the treatment. I took the news as if I had been punched between the eyes. I saw the nurse mouthing the words. I heard the words being said. There was no connection with my brain. It could not be possible they were turning me away.

I felt myself take a step to the side. I felt my face flush with embarrassment. I was being judged not strong enough for treatment. Mixed emotions swirled through me. Anger conveyed displeasure at being turned away. Fear took hold of the fact I was no longer in control of his body. Rejection told me I was a failure.

Nothing like this had ever happened to me before. I had cancer. That was understood. I was having treatment. That was fine. There had been a bit of pain but I had seen that out. I was ready for the next stage. Now I was being told my body was not fit for it. I almost felt the tears of despair and frustration start before I took control.

"What happens now?" I asked.

"Oh, wait a few days. Give yourself a bit more time. We'll book you back in on Monday. That's four days, should be enough. It's not unusual, you know".

I mumbled my thanks, lifted my bag onto my shoulder and stumbled back out the door.

So now I had been in the bed for the past six hours. I had started my long relationship with Stephen, although not on such familiar first name terms at that stage. The blood wash was on a drip. Twenty four hours of that before medication proper. Then twenty four hours of that, with the wash still being dripped into my body. After that it was for as long as it took with the wash to get the blood counts to correct, safe levels.

Harry had gently told me that I would be in for as long as a week, although five days should be sufficient. Methotroxate was a powerful drug, and without the wash would eat up all my organs. It was imperative to ensure that did not happen. So I would be checked daily for blood counts. Only when they were all at safe levels would I be allowed off the drip, and home.

The other consequence of all that liquid being pumped into my body was that I would need to go to the toilet very frequently. In fact I gradually noticed I went every hour, on the hour. The pattern emerged as I marked up each bottle I filled. Even those were taken away to be measured and tested. A slight by product of the treatment could be that I would become diabetic, even if only temporarily. There seemed to be no end to the good news. There seemed to be no end to the consequences to be uncovered. It all appeared to be akin to any criminal investigation unravelling all the clues and consequences.

For now, though, it was my first night. Angie, the night duty nurse, was doing the rounds with the drugs trolley. She stopped at the end of my bed, studying my board.

"Have you had your Dom Perignon?" I thought I heard her say.

That was better! I had not realised champagne was part of the treatment. No wonder the NHS needed extra funding. I had heard all the old stories of how people in the past were often given bottles of stout, usually Mackeson, to aid recovery, but this was higher class.

"Champagne? That part of the treatment? Oh, no. Haven't had that."

Angie looked up from the board, bemused. Her brows furrowed for a second before she laughed. "No. Not Dom Perignon. Donperidone, your anti-sick pills"

What a disappointment. What could I have done with a bottle of champagne? The thought would come back to me some months in the future.

32

The North London riots of 1985, which saw the murder of P.C. Keith Blakelock, highlighted the confusion in operational command of organisations involved in any major incident requiring the involvement of the emergency services. Following that particular event Scotland Yard realised that the standard rank based command system was not sufficiently responsive to dealing with such circumstances. The Metropolitan Police created a flexible command structure to be used by all emergency services, and involving local authorities. In the majority of cases the police would have primacy, but in the event of such as a major fire the Fire Service would take command until the immediate situation was under control. Then it would revert to the police for the investigation stage.

The system became known as the Gold-Silver-Bronze Command Structure. Bronze indicated the insight command, usually someone with control of all resources at the point of the incident, and based directly at that site. Silver covered the tactical management of an incident. Usually that would be remote from the site, but where information and resources could be co-ordinated, and deployed. Silver Command has the authority to deploy additional resources and would normally handle upward and downward briefings. Gold Command would normally only be declared if an incident required a strategic response.

The closeness of the police station to Bath Spa invited Bronze and Silver to exist in close proximity, albeit that Detective Superintendent Steve Chalmers who had direct responsibility for such investigations had to move into hastily prepared accommodation from his normal location. He quickly organised the needs of the investigation and established direct links to the wider intelligence sites operating in London, and Gold Command at Avon and Somerset Police Headquarters in Portishead, Bristol.

Gold Command was vested with Deputy Chief Constable James Lawson. His view of the situation went beyond the immediate investigation of what had happened. His concern spread to what could be a danger in the immediate future.

Thousands of people would be packing into Bath for the Festival opening. The risk of a repeat bombing was palpable. That possibility saw him striding into Bath Council Chambers at 10 o'clock that Friday morning to be met by the looks of the seven people already there. That seven comprised the Leader of the Council, the Deputy Leader who had responsibilities including commerce and marketing, three other cabinet members whose concerns included community safety, development and regeneration, leisure and culture, as well as transport and highways. All were relevant matter to the event that day. Also there was the Chief Executive.

He knew them all from various occasions of less serious natures than this. He could appreciate their looks of trepidation, hostility, defiance, anger and discontent long before he spoke.

The seventh person he had not met before. He was introduced as Daniel Ortaga, Director of the Musical Festival, and whose work was in jeopardy.

The Festival had enjoyed its golden jubilee just a few years before, following its inauguration in 1948. History had it that Bath had a strong musical tradition as far back as Queen Elizabeth 1's time, but more firmly established by the involvement of Beau Nash in the early eighteenth century. With its initial success the festival was taken over by the city. The Bath International Music Festival had become renowned for its quality and diversity, with many leading musicians show casing their talents in the historic buildings of the Pump Room, Assembly Room and Abbey, as well as a multitude of other venues. Spectacular events over the years had included a famous collaboration between Yehudi Menuhin and Ravi Shankar. The Three Tenors of Domingo, Carrerras and Pavarotti had also performed.

For such productions the quality and status of the Director required to be considerable. Daniel Ortaga had the musical pedigree, qualifications and professional recognition to set ever higher standards than the festival had previously known.

"You will realise that following the incident at Bath Spa yesterday I am concerned over the opening of the festival today. I believe there is a high risk in persevering with tonight's concert. It is my recommendation that the event be cancelled."

The reaction was immediate. There was consternation. It would be the downfall of the festival forever. It would be a travesty for the city. It would not be just a financial loss for the day, that weekend, but forever. There was no reason to link what happened last night to the festival. That was just scaremongering.

The debate became a six against one verbal boxing match. Every point raised by the six was countered by the one's response on public safety.

Daniel Ortaga listened carefully to what was being said. He realised that the Deputy Chief Constable was absolutely right in his concern. He also appreciated the fears of the council members. He had his own loyalties to the festival, its performers and audience. As the two sides drew breath he spoke for the first time.

"The concert is due to start at six this evening. I

believe I can adjust the programme to start an hour later. I also believe we can keep the audience out until six, and that one hour will be sufficient to get everyone in. Mr. Lawson, is there any chance that time will allow your investigation to establish any real danger to the festival? If there is, or you still feel there is too high a risk, we will cancel. However, to do so now would be very damaging."

All eyes swung to James Lawson. The expressions had changed. The anger, the despair had gone. Now they expressed hope, pleading and reconciliation. The risk could be immense. The responsibility was intense. Lives and futures had to be considered.

There was no assurance that last night had any linkage to this evening. If it did not that would be a civic disserve. If it did, and there were severe consequences, the repercussions would be traumatic.

"I will, very reluctantly, accede to your wishes. We will meet here at six o'clock. No audience will be allowed in the venue until we have met. You will provide sufficient resources to support a complete search of the venue this afternoon by our trained officers. And there is one other condition. Your stewards will ensure there is a minimum clearance of one hundred yards around the whole venue. I do not want any gatherings too close by."

So the dye was cast, but the chances of the concert taking place had paled, even in the eyes of the most hopeful.

33

"Morning boss, what can I do?" I worked hard to make my voice sound bright and energetic, even though the effort almost had me in a sweat.

I could see Ian Welsh groaning inwardly. I could see him thinking, "Can't this bloody Scotsman not put away his stubborn pride for just one day? There's enough going on without him to think about. He's not fit for the pace of what was going on. True, He's only been back for a week, or so, doing routine paperwork and some review work. He's done a lot of surveillance in his time, though. Maybe there was something he could do. If it keeps him quiet, and he thought he was helping another pair of eyes researching the CCTV footages would not go amiss". I could see it all flicker across his face.

"Actually, something right up your street! We've called in all the CCTV footage from the station, bus station, shopping centre. Everywhere. We've been through it but no joy. Maybe you'll see something. We haven't picked out anything that looks funny. No individuals show up as likely bombers. We've got everyone from every station from here to Milford Haven, Portsmouth and London checking in case it was someone who came in by train. Take them and see if you can spot anything. You've got the background. Everything's fitted up down the bottom room. You get tired, you tell me. Right?"

I nodded, smiled and turned away quickly to mask my disappointment. Surveillance, observation jobs just kept coming back to me. There was no point bitching about it. At least I would be doing something worthwhile looking at a screen. It had to be better than daytime television. I had had enough of that over the past few months, so watching repeats on a screen was no new experience to me.

34

Every month followed the same pattern. A pre visit for checks and to collect my tablet prescriptions. The start of the tablets before attending the ward. A full day of treatment by intravenous drip finishing with the dubious pleasure of the intrathecal.

The main difference was that each month my physical condition worsened. The first visit left me with no immediately recognisable reaction, or so I thought. I was quickly corrected.

Each month the cycle of treatment, decline in strength as the chemo did its work, the climb back to the nearest point to normality became more tortured. My energy levels quietly, insidiously deserted me. My reserves were reduced by each cycle. At the lowest point of each month I felt the strain of breathing as if I was atop Mount Everest, without the oxygen. It pained me to breathe. I felt as if I had aged by a hundred years. I also found that I did not just lose weight, at times I put it on so much I felt like the Michelin Man. It was the steroids that caused that.

My diet changed. I could no longer tolerate yoghurt in my mouth. The thought of drinking tea made me heave. Red wine became totally repugnant, at all times. I was thankful that in the good weeks I could still manage a glass of cold white wine. It must have been the different enzymes that made the difference!!

Coffee became addictive, but only secondary to grapefruit flavoured water. How I stumbled on that I was never quite sure. Perhaps Jimsi, a great water drinker, had brought it in. Maybe it had been someone else. Whoever it was had done me a big favour. It did have to be cold, straight out of the 'fridge. It had become my nectar.

I thought I had, at least, gained some insight into a woman's taste as she went through pregnancy.

Not everything was bleak. After four months a second scan failed to show any signs of the lymphoma. The treatment would be constrained to just six months. The neck pain was never repeated.

Harry had looked mildly embarrassed when told about the experience. "Ah! I'm sorry. If you remember when we gave you the injection we took some fluid out of your spine first to make room for what we had to inject. Obviously we took out too much. That's what caused the pain. It would have taken a few days to correct".

"Don't I bloody know it", I thought magnanimously, glad I would not go through that experience again.

35

"This is the twelve o'clock news from the BBC.

Scotland Yard say there is no breakthrough in the Bath Station bombing.

Chaos on the M6 as a lorry sheds its load of timber over the road.

Immigration figures cause another call for stricter controls.

Scotland Yard has released another statement on the investigation into the bombing at Bath Station. There has been no indication of why the bomb was placed. However, there is a claim that forensic examinations are beginning to illustrate how the bombing was carried out. From that it is hoped to identify groups that may be involved.

There has also been a telephone call to the BBC by an individual claiming to speak on behalf of the Animal Rights Movement. Code words indicate the call was authentic. The call claimed that the Movement had absolutely no involvement with the bomb. An assurance was given that the Movement does not take unilateral actions involving innocent people. Its actions only ever target those involved in cruelty towards animals, or who seek to profit from them.

A lorry has caused chaos…"

36

The clock ticked so slowly. The minute hand did not seem to move at all. Time did not seem so much as to pass, but be in suspension.

It was six o'clock. The blood counts had come back. Everything was fine. I could go home. That was the end of my third treatment of Methotroxate. Only this time I was not going home beyond a quick stop over to collect fresh clothing for a week or so. I was to stay with Jimsi and Niki. My sister could not come down from Scotland this time so Jimsi had insisted I stay with them.

The past six days had been as prolonged a period as I could remember. The first day I could take. The second, with the medication, was essential. Thereafter all I could do was wait, wash, eat, read and pee. It came to something when I began to bet with myself on whether I would fill the urine bottle with more, or less, than the time before.

Now I was packed, dressed and eager to go. I fully realised that I was going to feel awful again in a few days, that I would be more than happy to get back into bed and sleep more than a few hours away each day. That was always part of the deal, but it was on my terms, not within the four walls of the ward where I was not in control.

Not for the first time I counted my blessings. I had family and friends who looked out for me. I often wondered about those not so fortunate. Those who were reluctant to go to the doctor still bemused me. Those who had no doctor increasingly mystified me. I wondered about such as the homeless. They had no roots so where would they go for diagnosis? Who would look after them if they were in my situation?

There were so many questions, but so few answers.

I constantly considered myself lucky compared to others. Against that I had come to realise I was not immortal. There had been scares like the night with Barry, but that had been an external factor. This was from within. This was my body failing me. I was not old enough for that. It dawned on me I should make more of my life, enjoy more. There was no need to go wild. Just make more of what I had, like the car.

37

I saw the car soon after the surveillance had been set up. It was parked just in sight to any viewing customers. It was almost as if it was an embarrassment to the showroom. She was an old lady who did not meet the sexy demands of the modern day. Yet I saw her, and loved her at first sight.

The showroom was suspected of being the centre of drug dealing. It was a distribution point, or thought to be. Showroom was a bit of a grandiose description for a second hand car forecourt run from a rundown portacabin, in a far from salubrious area. In fact it was downright rough.

Against that the car was beautiful, to me, if to no one else.

The days went by. The log of observations filled. The evidence mounted. It was only a matter of time before the warrants would be issued. There was no knowing what would happen to the car. It could disappear forever.

I took time out to do some research. I had gone down to Halfords and browsed through the car manuals. That was the way in those days before household computers and search engines. Then I found it: A Rover P5B. What a car it was. What a beauty. Solid. Simple. It was too heavy for the modern flash, trash market. This was a car of substance: real bumpers, door handles where they were supposed to be, made of metal, no plastic involvement. Real leather seats. Real wood panelling. It was opulence at a manageable price from a bygone age. As I looked at the car I realised she was registered in 1971. She was over 20 years old, but she was gorgeous. I wanted her more than I had ever wanted anything.

So I did the unthinkable. I waited until I had a day off duty and went in to buy her. The deal was good and quick. I had her long before the raid was authorised.

Now, another dozen years on, she lay in a garage I had invested in for her when I moved to Bath. That had been a sound investment, not just for her, but for me. If I ever sold the garage I could buy a house in many parts of the country with those proceeds alone.

I was no mechanic but she was so simple to maintain I could do a lot of it myself. There was no computer diagnostics, just good old fashioned points, plugs, and tuning. Anything difficult and I had a horde of mechanics begging me to let them work on her. They all loved her, too.

Even the radio suited me. Two buttons: one for on/off, the other to tune into stations.

Oh, the comfort! Maybe that was why it had become a ministerial car for so long. Perhaps it had been part of the old "Buy British" policy, which had slipped into political incorrectness as a consequence of European Council membership. I was never sure. More recently I had heard that the Queen had owned an Arden green Rover P5 B Saloon which was on display at the Heritage Motor Centre. Mine was of a maroon hue which only got me abuse from those that knew me for being a poor man's "Morse". I never minded. Different car, different police force, different detective.

I had treated her badly in that for all I loved her, took care of her, tended to her every need, I spent too little time enjoying life with her. She was locked away for months at a time. Not that I was above saving the Road Tax by officially putting her "off the road" for the winter months. From now on they would take to the road more often. She was a classy lady. I would find out about vintage car clubs, put her on display. She could become a film star! Regardless, we would go out together more. Maybe Karen could be persuaded to join us.

Although I had names for some of my earlier cars I had never named her. Now, as I thought about it , it seemed to fit , that as an old lady I would enjoy driving Miss Daisy. Daisy she became, even though I knew that was less than original. She was getting on and now I was no longer sure what I had in front of me. The fifty per cent factor indicated I enjoy the pleasure now.

38

She came into the ward like a hurricane. She was five foot five inches of bristling energy. Carrot red hair bounced around her head, but not beyond the edge of her collar. Her green eyes gave truth to the stereotype of an Irish colleen, substantiated by the hint of an accent which identified her Hibernian birth. Questions and commands issued from her before the door finished closing behind her, and long before she arrived at the desk.

That was my introduction to Sister Karen Gillen, the matriarch and driving force of the William Budd Ward. I was enthralled by her energy, her commitment and sheer drive to ensure that every patient got all that they needed.

In all the time I went in and out of the hospital I never once saw her less than in control of any situation. She seemed to know everyone, and everything about everyone. No matter if a nurse was distracted from a drip change to deal with something else Karen would look up, determine what was going on and keep things running. It mattered not whether it was in the Daycare area, down the corridor in the Chemo Suite, or the main ward when she took time in there, she always had her finger on the metaphoric pulse.

I mused over her age. Possibly early to mid thirties, I thought, but never sought to verify my suspicions. I certainly would not ask anyone else. The dangers of appearing in the least interested were too much to contemplate. Maybe she was involved with someone else, though where she would find the time I did not know. She wore no rings on her left hand. Given my state of health it was hardly the right time to get interested in anyone else.

She would know better than me what fifty percent

survival expectation amounted to. Maybe one day I would get bolder, but not for a long time.

Over the months we got to speak more often. She knew what I did and the parody of us both dealing with different ailments in society gave substance to those brief interludes. I worried about her pace of working, never seeming to have a proper lunch, only eating sandwiches as she worked on. I rebuked her constantly but she just laughed it off, and carried on regardless. She always came back for more, and there was always a sparkle in her eye as we verbally jousted.

As time went by and I thought more and more about re-assessing my life, taking more time to enjoy its pleasures, the idea of having a companion on my spins with old Daisy started to take form.

39

By lunch time I had scanned through all there was to see. I had drawn up a list of viewing sights, cross matched times and drawn up a list of priorities to review again.

Patience and diligence. It had been drummed into me. Whole investigations could come to nothing because of missing that single act, that single moment that demonstrated the link. Diligence was not a good working partner with tiredness, and I was tired. My eyes were strained. My concentration was becoming frayed. I could not keep going. I needed a break.

I rubbed my eyes. I massaged my cheeks feeling the fine downy hair that used to be harsh bristle before the chemotherapy. At least there was something there. When had I last shaved? Five days ago? It did not matter just now. I needed a cup of coffee and something to eat, but could not face the smell of the canteen. I would go out and get something at Marks and Spencers, something light and refreshing. I could pick up a coffee on the way back.

The fresh air jolted my senses, so that despite myself I was glad to get back to the warmth of the room. So much so I slept for half an hour without any knowledge of drifting into unconsciousness. I shook myself awake and reached for the tapes again. For the next two hours I watched, scanned, sifted and selected. Then I was down to two tapes, and the connection between them.

40

My view of life brightened on the day of the bone marrow tests. I was to be at the William Budd Ward of the RUH for one o'clock. The naming of the ward interested me. I always liked to know the derivation of things, and place names were particularly intriguing. I guessed it must be named after some well known figure in the cancer world. Little did I know I would come to accept the ward as some form of second home over the next six months, and be able to find out a little more about the man whose name had been given to it.

On the due date I found my way to the ward. I entered the hospital by the main entrance. That was the new main entrance, with its modern design of high glass roof and plenty of space. I followed the signs along corridors until I found myself in a part of the hospital that was single storey, red brick construction of World War Two vintage. It was very much like a number of similar structures in the city built on the principle of a long corridor with adjoining arms all the way down, on both sides. This one seemed to be the only one I could think of as performing the task it was built for. All the others had long since become offices for the Ministry of Defence.

I reported to the ward's main reception, and was directed to the day care area. Once there I was ushered into the bed section, advised to make myself comfortable, and "wait for the doctor". The wait was worthwhile. First to appear was Julie, the nurse who had seen me on arrival. Middle aged; well padded she had the appearance of a good old fashioned country girl. Just behind her was someone of a different world.

She was a vision. She was tall, slim, elegant, with long auburn hair flicked behind her ears. Tanned skin and large dark eyes that seemed to draw me in like as a drowning man in a deep pool of water.

"Hullo. I'm Emily. I'm one of the registrars here". She went on about other things as I struggled to get over the notion that I needed to be considerably younger to make any sort of impression on her, to match the one she had made on me. I gradually surfaced from the deep pool recognising I was there for treatment. This was not an arrangement made by some blind dating agency. Shame though that might be.

I sat, almost open mouthed, as her words began to be more meaningful. Firstly, I was to go to the X-ray department to have a scan. She patiently explained the abbreviations stood for Computerised Tomography, which simply referred to the technology of the equipment. I would need to drink some liquid "dye" before that actually happened. That scan would pinpoint anything internally. Then I would come back for a bone marrow extraction from my hip bone. I nodded my understanding, hoping my silence would be interpreted as concern for my situation, not for acting like a lovelorn teenager.

The scan, itself, took about fifteen minutes passing through a giant, open drum like chamber. It was absolutely painless, other than the taste of the drink. The whole process, though, took well over an hour to get back to the ward.

When I got back Julie and Emily were quickly by my side with a small operating pack. Emily looked concerned. "How do you feel about the options of how we do this? We can knock you out which would ensure you would feel nothing, but leave you a little unsteady afterwards. Or, we could just give you a local".

My eyebrows raised in question. "Why? Do

you think I'm too old to take the pain?"

"Not at all. It's not a matter of being too old. Rather, you are still relatively young". Pity about the relatively, I thought. "If you look around you'll see most people in here are older than you. Most have just had a local. As the body ages the bones soften and it is easier to get a small core sample without causing distress. You're bones will still be hard, so it will be more painful. The compromise may be to start with a local and if it gets too sore to top it up".

I looked around and could see that everyone looked at least twenty years older than me. "Let's try the local to start", I offered, with more conviction than I felt.

"Right. As we get ready could you get up on the bed, pull down your trousers over your hips, and lay on your side".

As I lay there I felt Emily's hands gently pass over the top of my buttocks kneeding the skin. Satisfied she had found the right spot she said"You'll feel a little prick". I clenched my teeth against any response. She was referring to the injection, nothing else. I felt her working behind me as Julie came into view. She talked to me. I responded knowing she was trying to distract me. All the time I was aware of the needle, but it was never going to be too sore.

When it was over it was explained that when the tests had been analysed I would get the results in a few days. I was getting used to hearing that expression.

41

I tried to read the letter again. I had lost count of the times I had tried to read it. I had read all the words but they had only registered in isolated groups, or singly. I had not been able to comprehend the letter as an entity.

It was no better this time. Nor would it ever be. It would always be a kaleidoscope of words and feelings with different emphasis each time I ever read it.

Now the most salient words that I could focus on were "biopsy confirms a diffuse large B cell lymphoma" "Lymph mode in the right oxilla and bilateral lower lobe atilectasis and consolidation of the lungs"

"is at least stage III lymphoma"

"5 years overall recovery rate of approximately 50%"

"it is potentially a curable malignancy"

Only potentially?

"Initial response rate to this chemotherapy is around 65-70% with an overall survival of patients in his category at 50%!

Somehow the written word seemed much more desolate than the sympathetic tone when I had been told. After all the tests I had been called in for a consultation to Dr Knightley's clinic in the William Budd Ward.

When I arrived I was lead into a consulting room already occupied by two people. One was the delectable Emily, the other was a tall man with black hair swept back in the style of an old matinee idol. His handsome features were accentuated by the brown skin of his Indian birth.

The doctor rose in welcome, extending his hand. "Hello, please take a seat. I am Dr Probaharan of Dr Knightley's team. Call me Harry, everyone else does. It is so much easier. This is my colleague Emily, who you have previously met.

I smiled tightly to both. It was almost too hard to smile. For some reason I was again aware of a dark chasm opening before me. In almost any other circumstance I would have found it very easy to smile, especially for Emily.

Harry looked at me earnestly. "You will have no doubt gathered that we have good reason to want to talk to you. We now have the results of the tests and the scan that have been done on you. We have found that you have lymphoma. The scan shows shadows in both lungs and while they are not absolutely conclusive we are taking the view that the lymphoma is on both sides of your diaphragm. That increases the score and therefore the seriousness with which we must approach the treatment. We are suggesting most strongly that you be treated with radiotherapy and chemotherapy.

There was a slight pause as Harry looked at the consternation, confusion and apprehension in the face before him. "The treatment is typical although we will make the mix specific for you. It is a standard approach for your condition. To put it into every day terms I am afraid I have to tell you that you do have cancer.

Soon after that the colours began to spiral in front of my eyes.

42

I remembered leaving the room. I would always remember that. It was a strange feeling that had enveloped me. It was almost three dimensional in that it was as if my senses had separated from my body and I watched myself from across the corridor.

The two aspects of my being started out towards the exit. Slowly, step by step, they moved closer until by the time I reached the door I was one again.

A deep breath, a blink of the eyes and a squaring of my shoulders would have been the only signs of my understanding. There was no point feeling sorry for myself. I just had to accept the situation and get on with things.

Harry had carefully explained why this condition was high on the risk scale. The findings lead to scorings which gave me a 5 year overall survival rate of 50%. The proposed treatment had a response rate of 65-70% with an overall survival for patients in this category of 50%.

Not great betting odds I had thought. No more than evens, really. Still the 65-70% sounded a little bit better.

The treatment was called "R-CHOP" Again my imagination started. "Getting the chop doesn't sound good" flashed through my mind.

Harry patiently continued "I know this all sounds very strange to you but the terminology merely describes the drugs the course of chemotherapy consists of.

Another jolt of reality hit me. Chemotherapy wasn't just chemotherapy; it was a lot more complicated than that. I had not known that but doubted if many did if they were not involved.

"Before you go we'll give you some literature to

take away. One will describe all the drugs in CHOP. The section R is for Rituximab, another drug we feel it sensible to add to give a greater option for you. We will give you six to eight courses along with intrathecal chemotherapy which we will alternate each month between Methotrexate and Cytorabine."

The weight of information, the complications of drug names, was starting to make me wilt. A fog was descending over me. I shot out of that into clear light when I heard what Harry said next, "You will understand that the intrathecal treatment is given by injections into your spine". "No", I thought, "I hadn't". The thought of a needle being pushed into my spine made me feel hot and cold almost simultaneously. I was immediately scared I could finish up in a wheel chair if anything went wrong.

Almost as if he was telepathic Harry continued, "Only fully trained and certified staff can give you the intrathecal, so there is no need to worry.

Between the second and third, fourth and fifth treatments we will take you in for a few days, up to a week, to give you high doses of Methotrexate intravenously. Each month you will have to come in for a consultation a few days before your treatment date to assess your condition, check your weight to allow us to calculate the strengths to give you and collect your prescriptions for these medicines you start before coming in. At the end of the Chemotherapy you will also have radiotherapy on your testis".

By then my body and mind were beginning to separate. I barely heard being told I would lose my hair, possibly suffer extremes of nausea, suffer mouth ulcers, that I had to ensure no exposure to the sun or to the cold, that I would be easily exhausted. The warning that the treatment could well affect my ability to have children did raise a small, sardonic smile. Now that did up the ante from merely having a testicle removed.

The pile of literature was finally placed in my hands and I passed through the door to start that long walk down the corridor.

43

It was lunchtime when he got back to the house. The bicycle ride back from the University was almost all along a flat terrain, but just the few slight inclines had pulled at his leg muscles. His breathing became ragged when before all this he would not have even registered any effort. His strength was clearly fading.

Despite that he was inwardly cheerful. He recovered the bottles, watches and corks before settling down to his task. The watches were all primed for 10 o'clock. He did think about varying some but that might mean them being ineffective if people moved in the wrong direction for his plans. It would be better having them all synchronised. He carefully married them up and slipped each one home.

Satisfied with that stage he took a sharp kitchen knife out of the cutlery drawer to pare the corks to fit into the necks of the bottles. The effort was beyond his belief. Just cutting cork and pushing each into a bottle was causing the sweat to drip from his face again. By the time he had finished his hands were trembling.

He poured a cup of cold water and leaned, gasping, against the kitchen sink as he drank it.

All he had to do then was cut off the tops of the corks, tidy up, get the picnic basket out, pack it with the bottles, have some lunch, book a taxi, put his clothes in the wash basket, set the alarm for 4 o'clock, and have a sleep.

He intended to be fully prepared and rested for the night's concert.

44

I shook myself awake and reached for the tapes.

I watched them again.

I saw the tall, blond haired man walk into the station.

I saw the tall, blond haired man walk out of the station just a few minutes later, parting from two very small, dark haired ladies who were obviously from the Far East.

Why meet them, then leave them?

I swapped tapes.

I saw the tall, blond man arrive on the platform. He had a ticket but had not seemed to have stopped to buy one. Either he had purchased one previously, had a return ticket to somewhere, or had a season ticket.

I scribbled a note. Check ticket sales.

The man made no attempt to board the train, or display any interest in getting on. Rather he seemed to be waiting, looking for someone.

The two young ladies were struggling with their luggage. He moved over to them, clearly offering to help. Their expressions reflected their delight and admiration for this chivalrous, handsome young man. He adjusted something in his shoulder bag, picked up two of their suitcases, and they all moved towards the exit.

Puzzled, I punched the eject button and swapped tapes.

I watched the man enter the station. I watched the group join the queue for a taxi. I saw the man wave goodbye and move away from the front of the station.

I watched the sequence again and again. Something was not right. Something was happening, but I could not spot what it was. There was also a growing familiarity about the man.

Again I watched the man go in the stat
ion. I saw the shoulder bag swing by his side.

I watched the man leave the station. I saw the shoulder bag swing out as he leaned over to put down the suitcases. I saw him shrug his shoulders with that exertion.

I saw the man walk away, but there was no shoulder bag!

I watched it again. I saw it again.

I repeated the process.

That was it! The shoulder bag was shrugged off as the suitcases were put down. It was left there and the man moved away.

It was deliberate. It was planned. There was no way anyone could not know they had just lost a shoulder bag in that sort of situation.

My breath left me in one long stream. My eyes closed. My shoulders hunched. "This must be it. This is how it was done", I thought. The time on the tapes showed 16.19.

But who was it? The gnawing started to grow. I watched again, and again, concentrating on the face of that tall, blond man.

I knew the face. I was positive of that.

45

I knew the face, but from where?

Think!

Think!

Slow down. Think logically.

Where?

I reviewed my old cases. No matches.

I thought through social occasions. No matches.

I thought through sporting events. No matches.

I scanned my memory of local news events. No matches.

It was so close. I knew it was. It just would not come to me.

I watched the clip again. I watched the walk. I felt himself mimic the movements. There was a slight, self confident swagger about the shoulders. Somehow, from somewhere I already knew it.

I knew the man, for crying out loud!

Who was he?

I closed my eyes. In the darkness my mind and memory travelled again. Flying high, speeding, gliding, swooping into the recesses of my brain. False dawns came and went. It was so close. I knew it, I knew it.

Then it was in front of me. I saw the walk. I saw the movement across the room. I saw the women turn to look admiringly at the man. I saw him in what had virtually become my second home. I saw him in William Budd Ward.

46

I was dozing. The morning was sunny and the heat through the window had brought on a spell of lethargy. It had been another disturbed night. The morning routines of breakfast and ward cleaning had finished. My medication was up to date. There was a lull which brought about a seductive invitation to close my eyes.

"Well, well, well, what have we here? What you been up to, Cocker?"

The voice came from the door sparking recognition in my memory. My eyes fought to open and focus. There was only one person that ever called me "Cocker". Bob Smith had pretty well adopted me when I joined the Bath police team. We had worked together on and off for a number of years until Bob retired some two years previously. In turn I wondered if it really could be Bob, and what on earth possessed him to be here.

My eyes gradually opened, widened, and eventually focused on the figure now moving round my bed, pushing a tea trolley.

"Bob! What are you doing here?"

"Serving tea, do it two days a week. The wife got me involved after I retired. I quite enjoy it."

It slowly came back to me. Ann Smith had long been a Friend of the R.U.H. doing voluntary work for the hospital. Obviously Bob had been recruited.

Bob was not in a hurry. He was almost finished his round and the tea could not stew any stronger than it already was. So he settled in for an account of my condition, which was given without embellishment.

"So that was it. Started by going to Oncology, then when the results of the biopsy came out got transferred to Haematology, here, and now going through chemotherapy."

"Well, you did the right thing getting it seen to quickly. I've seen too many come in here that have left it too late. It's heartbreaking, and mostly down to sheer stupidity, or a fear of facing up to it. Trouble is if you leave it too long it gets a stronger hold of you and it's more difficult to treat. People can only take strong enough chemo to kill off the cancer if they have the strength to stand up to it. The more hold it has the weaker it makes them, so the chemo mix has to be weaker. The weaker the mix the harder it is to kill off the cancer. Catch 22. You've got to be brave and face it head on."

Bob eventually had to leave, but he did so with a promise to call back whenever he was doing his turn.

The name of Cocker was one that simultaneously amused and irritated. Bob had bestowed it on me through some strange logic that as I had come down from London I was a Cockney, therefore a Cocker. No amount of protestation that I really came from the North of Scotland ever held any sway.

47

The naming of the William Budd Ward had intrigued me from the very start. As it was the "cancer ward" I had developed a theory that there had to be an association with a cancer specialist, or something of that ilk.

During one of old Bob's tea runs we had been chatting and I mentioned my interest. Bob had looked nonplussed for a second. "You know, I've been doing this for two years and I've never given it a thought. Now you mention it there must be a story. Leave it to me. I'll find out. I haven't done any detective work for a long time. Thanks for that".

I thought over Bob's words with a mixture of mild irritation and amusement. Irritation that I had wanted to find out for myself, but accepting there was no immediate prospect of being able to do anything about it. The amusement came from the little spring in Bob's step, the lift of his head. I could see that Bob had set himself a mission. The more I thought about it the more amused, and pleased, I became, while the irritation melted away. The smile was still on my lips as I drifted off to sleep once more.

Time came and went, and it was not until my next long visit that the subject came up again. Bob bounced into the ward, his face wreathed in a broad smile.

"Well, Cocker, it's not quite the whole story. And it's not quite what you thought. I've hunted everywhere, asked everyone I could get hold of. Been through the hospital records.

Dr. William Budd was about a bit before cancer became known as it is now. Seems he was born in North Tauton in Devon in 1811. He studied medicine in London, Paris and Edinburgh. Nothing but the best. Seems to have turned up in Bristol about 1841 working at St. Peter's Hospital and the Infirmary, where he was heavily involved with care during the typhoid and cholera epidemics. There was no cure at the time but he sort of specialised and identified the dangers of water borne disease. He became a real crusader for clean water supply and was an early director of the Bristol Waterworks Company. Seems he had a hard fight against the medical establishment but when the 1866 cholera epidemic got to Bristol the much reduced death rate in the city, compared to elsewhere, vindicated his theories.

He became one of the city's most distinguished physicians. There's a plaque at 899, Park Street in Bristol commemorating him. Guess he lived there.

The only thing I can't find is the link as to why this ward should have his name. He doesn't seem to have any link with Bath, nor with cancer.

Best I could do. Not complete, but it was good fun finding out."

We mulled it over. It was slightly disappointing not get a full answer, but no disaster. The thought that there was no relationship seemed strangely apt. After all, so much cancer had no discernible connection to how, and why, it was there, but it was.

48

It was another long night. Even my light was out. I had given up trying to pass the time. It just seemed to be standing still. I had concluded I would just relax, and let my body float away. A little bit like transmeditation, I thought. Deep down I knew I did not really know what that was all about.

I had read about it somewhere, sometime. Empty the mind seemed to be the first step. Fall into peaceful tranquillity. Perhaps that would be as good as the produce of the Glen of Tranquility: that fine Glenmorangie malt whisky. Not Spey, of course, but more than acceptable for all that. Stop! Too much thinking. Start again.

Then I heard the trolley rumbling up the corridors. Shoes slithered over the vinyl tiled floor in an attempt to keep any noise down. Material rustled as legs pummelled beneath crisp uniform skirts. Urgent whispered questions, instructions, quietly echoed through the rooms.

"Something bad for someone", I thought. The idea of emptying my mind was a lost cause. It was not the first time this type of interruption had happened. Maybe it was just someone being sick. That did not explain the need for the trolley.

One time before I had been on the point of asking the nurse who came in to change my drip, sometime after the event. One look at her face, far removed from her normal cheery countenance, stilled the question long before it reached my lips.

Another time I had not needed to ask. The girl in the room across the corridor just was not there in the morning.

49

I sat still trying to rationalise my thoughts. I did not hear the call from the door. I was oblivious to all about me. I was totally unaware of anything beyond the pictures that framed in my mind. I did not even see the office I was sitting in. All I saw was the man walking past me, but in the hospital.

I was shocked back to reality by a hand falling on my shoulder, and a voice very close to my ear saying in a very measured tone "Detective Sergeant. Far be it from me to have to tell you, for the third time in the past ten seconds, but go home! I told you yesterday. Now I'm telling you again. You're shot. You didn't even know I've been speaking to you. I shouldn't have allowed you to stay this long. Now go!"

"But, boss......"

"Don't argue. I'm telling you to go home. You've been here long enough. You've watched everything we have and not come up with anything. We're all getting tetchy. This whole thing makes no sense. No motive. No clues. We're all under pressure. The D.S. is under pressure. He's applying pressure. As the man in charge of this operation he needs results. Nothing is breaking. I don't need the worry that you're the only thing that is going to break up. So just go home and rest".

"But..."

"No! Go!"

My mind reeled. I knew I had something to offer. Not something in the sense of my training and experience but something real, tangible, relevant to the case. Or I thought I had. It dawned on me I had not had time to explore my vision. I did not have enough to argue with. My head went down. I could almost taste frustration. Very quietly I said "Okay, boss".

I felt a sympathetic clap on my shoulder, then I was

on my own. I sighed as I raised myself from the chair. I looked at my watch. The time was 4.05: almost twenty four hours since the start of that misguided run out into the street.

50

It was one of those interminable days. The outlook was grey. The rain had been unrelenting. I had no wish to go out. It would not have mattered if I had. I did not have the energy.

My sister had been down looking after me for a week but she had left to fly back to Scotland that morning. All the washing and ironing was up to date .The 'fridge and cupboards were fully stocked. There was nothing to do, but I did not have the inclination to even think about that anyway.

Time stood still again.

The questions kept coming back.

How did I get the cancer?

Why did I get it?

Why the way I had got it?

When did I get it?

At least I had some comfort with the last one. By all accounts it had not been too long ago. I had acted on a relatively early sign and that had been to my benefit. A 50/50 chance was better than 60/ 40 against.

I had learned that I had not suddenly developed cancer. The cells were always there, just kept in check. So my initial thinking that some of my body cells had suddenly been corrupted was wrong. I had compared it to the corruption, and insidious conversion, of people to terrorism, and the common practice of bombing that blew away the good and the innocent.

Rather it was just waiting for a chance to break out and take over. Poor defences allowed that to happen. I just did not know how my defences had let me down, and no one could tell me. I had been over this so often, but was never any nearer an answer. It reminded me so much of those unsolved crimes. All centred around the same questions.

How?

When?

Where?

Who?

Somewhere along the line an answer to an unresolved question would be the key to the solution.

I unfolded the blanket lying on the settee. I stretched out along its length tucking the blanket under my chin. I drifted off to sleep. There was nothing better to do that day, nor would there be for the next few days.

51

As I reached the foot of the stairs I was overtaken by a young constable.

"Hey, Deek. How you doing?"

"God, Sarge. Better me than you by the look of you"

"Young man, that's no way to speak to a senior officer."

Derek Hailes was a bright young man. Tall, dark haired, with a slightly swarthy complexion he was a keen sportsman, who for whatever reason from his past was known throughout as Deek. It certainly was not as a derivation of geek. Over the past couple of years we had struck up a rapport through our mutual involvement in the rugby club.

"Maybe, but you're not looking great. You off home?"

I hesitated. I knew the answer should be a straight "yes", if I was to follow instruction, but the wheels were slowly grinding out an idea in my mind.

"Could be. No rush. As you say, I couldn't anyway. What are you doing?"

"Just the usual. Going out and about on the west side of town."

"Bingo", I thought. "Don't suppose you could give me a run out to the R.U.H., could you?"

Deek looked at me appraisingly. Something told him this was not right. He did not know why, but clearly something in my voice betrayed that it was more than a casual question. Yet there was no reason to feel it was anything untoward.

"Bit late for an appointment, isn't it?"

"Hospitals are open twenty four hours a day. Yes or no?"

"Okay, but you better not be in a hurry. The traffic will be hell."

I thought I would wait to see what the traffic was like before I asked about putting the blue light on.

52

Deek knew all the shortcuts, keeping away from the main roads, and we were soon on the Upper Bristol Road. Presently we were passing by the Royal Victoria Park, where preparations were still being carried out for the evening's concert. Then onto Newbridge Hill, heading steadily west before turning into Combe Park and onto the hospital.

"Deek. I need to see someone for a few minutes. It's not about me. I'll be honest with you. I'm doing something I'm not sure I should be doing, but I just have a feeling. I've been told to go home, but I just need to check out something to do with what happened last night. Can you hang around for me?" Deek glanced over very quickly, before bringing his eyes back to the traffic. I could see he was suddenly felt uncomfortable again. "How do you mean?" he asked.

"Maybe it's nothing but I've got to check out whether there's a link between someone I saw on the videos today and someone I've seen at the hospital. Just a few minutes." The last words were spoken in a whisper. There was no attempt to add suspense. It was just evidence, even to me, of obvious tiredness.

Deek clearly thought I was going too far, but if I felt I had to do what I had in mind, in the state I was in, there must be something to it. Again he agreed.

53

I had been running a bit tight for my appointment time as I pushed open the outer doors at the end of the corridor from William Budd.

An elderly lady was sitting on one of the chairs in the small waiting area just inside the door. She looked up expectantly, hoping to see if it may be the person she was waiting for to take her home. Displaying no disappointment she smiled brightly at me. "Good morning. Lovely day, isn't it?" I smiled a reaction, agreeing it was. As I moved past her she stretched her arm out.

"Excuse me for saying so, but I do like your hat".

I stopped in mid stride, turning towards her, feeling my cheeks flush like a small boy with embarrassment. The hat had become one of the features of my defences. I had stuck religiously by the warnings that there had to be no risks of getting a cold, nor was there to be any exposure to the sun. Even on the warmest of days I had button downed long sleeves.

Today was a fine day but with a slight chill in the breeze so the hat was in use. There were not many days I did not wear it now. In fact I had got to like wearing it. I had bought it on a whim the previous year in Philadelphia when I had gone across to the United States with the family for my nephew's wedding. Bigger than a trilby, smaller than a Stetson, I always thought of it as my Indiana Jones hat. It had that look about it.

"Thank you" I managed to stammer, before she continued. "It has a touch of class about it. You don't see much real style nowadays".

I stayed with her, telling her how I had bought it, forgetting my concern for my time keeping. I was saved from being late by a call from the door for the lady.

As I walked up the corridor I realised I was walking straighter than before. My step had more bounce. I felt uplifted. Was that just a woman, or had an angel called on me? Just a few kind words and I felt so much better about life.

54

As the car turned into the hospital I told Deek to turn to the right and park outside the old building side door. The small car park there was almost empty.

"I'll be as quick as I can", I said, as I got out. I suddenly felt stiff. And a little light headed. I entered the building through the door where the lady had complimented me on my hat. There was no one there this time, but I touched the hat brim anyway. I started up the corridor but it took on the dimensions of a tunnel. It seemed no matter how far I walked I was making little progress. A dampness rose on my brow. My eyes were stinging. My lungs were performing in that laboured way that came to me after each chemo session.

Eventually I got to the ward. I entered main reception. It was deserted. I walked on through, struggling against the invisible ropes that someone had somehow looped over me and were using to hold me back. My whole body felt as if I was in a shower. I turned into the day care room. As I entered I saw a couple of the chairs were still occupied. I looked towards the desk. She was there.

"Karen?"

Her head snapped up. Her eyes expressed surprise at seeing me, but quickly gave way to concern over my appearance. "What's the matter? I thought we had seen the last of you in here. You look awful. Are you alright?"

I reached the desk. "Karen. I need to talk to you, but it's not about me. I need to ask you something. I need your help". I stopped, conscious that pairs of eyes were watching, pairs of ears listening. "Can we go into the back office?" As we retreated into that room, more of a storage room for case files, my hand went to my pocket. As Karen turned I held out my wallet to show my warrant card.

"This is police business. I need you to help me identify someone." I regretted I had not thought to go back and run off a photograph before coming, but it had not been planned. I saw the surprised register in her eyes.

"Just a little while ago this afternoon I was looking at CCTV footage and saw someone I'm sure I've seen here. I need to know who he is, even if only to........ check he is not involved." I struggled not to use the hackneyed phrase "eliminate from our enquiries". No doubt it would have been used often enough during the day on the news.

"I'm convinced I've seen him here – only once, maybe, and not too long ago. Tall, slim guy in his early twenties I would say. Blond hair. Good looking boy. Drew lots of glances from the ladies".

I saw her eyes widen. I saw the recognition flicker. "You know who it is, don't you?"

"I…. yes….but I can't. Patient conf… ". Her eyes drifted away from me.

I cut her short. "Karen. I haven't got time. I haven't got the energy to argue. All I can say is it is important. You'll know what happened yesterday? That's why I need to speak to this guy." Her hand flew to her mouth. Her eyes registered shock and alarm. Then, for the first time ever, I saw the uncertainty in her expression.

"I can't…!

"Please, Karen. I know about patient confidentiality. But I'm not asking for any details about him. Just who is he? Where can I find him?"

"I should ask for advice….."

"It's getting on for five o'clock. What chance is there? I need to know now. If there is any possibility he's involved who's to say he wont do it again, maybe soon. Look, don't tell me. Couldn't you just lay his file on the desk, bring him up on the screen. Anything that would allow me to see who he is, without you telling me."

I saw her eyes widen. The green seemed to soften as she considered the possibility. Then they dimmed with a form of resignation, before snapping back to their normal glint. I saw her visibly make up her mind. She transformed to the brisk, efficient Karen I had come to know. She wheeled away from me and marched to the computer. She tapped at the keyboard for a review of records. The screen flickered and transformed.

"There", she said looking at me. "I have to see to my patients"

I whispered my thanks. Relief, and pain over what I had forced her to go through, swept over me.

She turned away. I glanced at the screen. I noted the name and address. I left as quickly as I was able without inviting more attention from those enquiring eyes across the room.

It seemed less likely now that Karen would be joining me for that run with Miss Daisy.

55

By the time I got back to the car I was gasping.

"Everything okay?" I enquired of Deek, as I slumped into the passenger seat.

"Yeah. Just checked in that I am in the area. Nothing doing. Get your business done?"

"Mmmm. Need to go to Combe Down, urgently. Someone else to see. Can you get me there? I'll need to 'phone in what's happening. No point trying to go back through town. Go the long way and get the siren on."

If Deek felt it was getting too much he never showed it. Rather he seemed to like the prospects. A slight smile pulled at his lips as he started away, quickly switching on the emergency system. Something was going on. His passenger was definitely up to something. I may have looked like death but he knew something was driving me on. It had to be special to keep me going like this. If he just did the driving he would find out soon enough.

The car sped back down Combe Park. At the end it spun to the right into Newbridge Hill, leading away from the city centre. We passed the grand old houses set back in large gardens, some now less imposing than in days of yore, more posing than imposing. The traffic was reasonably light and easy to navigate through.

Turning onto the steep decline of Old Newbridge Hill brought the first potential hold up, with cars parked on both sides, and a queue waiting to join Newbridge Road. Drivers grudgingly gave ground. At the bottom of the hill Deek swept out into the main flow forcing cars on both sides to give way, again moving west and away from the city. He drove hard now, forcing more cars to give ground, sweeping over the river bridge and up to the traffic lights. Mercifully they were at green and he turned right again heading along the Bristol

Road.

Half a mile along he turned left at the roundabout, passing the Globe Inn. Up the hill, over and down, down to the base of Whiteway before the start of the long climb. We came to houses on the left marking the boundary of Bath, with open fields and rolling scenery to the right. Up and up the hill we climbed scattering cars like the chaff that would be in those fields in a few months time.

Onto the level passing the cemetery and crematorium Deeks eyes were fixed ahead measuring the next obstruction to their progress. Just for a second I allowed my eyes to wander and the thought passed through my mind that I could have made a final journey in there if things had not gone well for me.

On and on, the traffic getting heavier again as we moved into a more built up area. Deek was switching over the road and back. Culverhay School came and went. Another incline, climbing up Rush Hill, then onto Frome road. The road was narrow now, the traffic heavy and becoming obstructive as it was in turn held up by the traffic coming out of the centre up Wellsway. I noticed Deek's knuckles were turning white, the fingers tense round the driving wheel, but our progress did not falter. We screeched across the roundabout at the top of Wellsway bulleting along, mercifully past the time the road would have been blocked by doting mothers collecting offspring from the Fosseway Infant School. We shot across the double roundabout and onto Bradford Road.

Now past the worst of the traffic I punched the buttons of my mobile 'phone. The response was almost immediate. I did not waste time.

"Boss, I think I have the identity of the bomber. I'm on my way…" I stopped for a second. I did not want to get into a long conversation. "Sorry, you're breaking up. I need full back up and quickly". I gave the address. Then I switched the 'phone off. I did not want a call back.

"Do you know where that is?" I asked Deek. "Pretty well" was the answer.

We were heading into Combe Down. Quickly the M.O.D. site at Foxhill, where Jimsi had worked, was before us on the left. Immediately opposite was the Foresters, a public house where we had enjoyed a few pints after work. Neither registered as I concentrated on what may be in just a couple of minutes. "Cut the siren. No point warning him".

The top of Ralph Allen Drive was fast approaching. Past that we took the first right into Tyning Road at the Horseshoe pub. Luckily no one was coming the other way. I had not thought of it before but an accident of any sort at this stage could get us both into really serious trouble. "What the hell", I thought, "Bigger things to worry about".

Deek was already turning into Gladstone Place, and our destination was in front of us, a taxi at the front door.

56

The house was imposing in a quiet, understated way. Built of Bath stone more than a hundred years before, the colour had mellowed to a dark honey hue. There was a central porch extending from the front showing a large door. The eaves hung low giving a cottage effect magnified by the roses climbing the walls on both sides of the porch. Not that the house was a cottage. It was much larger than that. The semi circular driveway which swept from the gateway they entered by up to the house and round to a similar opening at the far end of the garden wall belied belonging to just a cottage.

I saw all that as Deek swept onto the drive. I saw the taxi at the house front and the tall figure coming out of the door. I saw the picnic basket in the man's right hand, the jerk of his head as he, in turn, saw the police car, and the break in his step.

Deek did not slow down until he had to, slewing the car to a stop with a shower of gravel. He was still turning the ignition key off as I was out the door and moving towards the tall man, with his right hand extended, showing my warrant card. Deek watched the scene for just a split second before he was moving himself. It was like watching an old detective film." Tom Stevens? Police. I would like to speak to you".

The impression of a film was reinforced by the man's appearance. He was dressed in a vaguely green linen suit, with a long silk scarf slung loosely round his neck, and a Panama hat which could not conceal the golden hair escaping from the back of his neck. Deek's first thought was that he looked a bit of a dandy on his way to the Festival concert. He was not to know how true that was.

By the time he got round the car I was asking the man to put down the basket. "Constable, would you take Mr. Steven's to the car, please. I'll need to speak to the taxi driver for a second". That individual was in his cab, mouth akimbo, and eyes bulging. He operated from the rank just a hundred yards from the police station and knew a lot of the officers, but had never seen anything like this. He saw me approaching in his wing mirror . As my face appeared at the window he suddenly realised he knew who it was, even if I did look very ill and colourless. I was one of his regular fares.

Before he had a chance to move I opened his door. "Sorry,Tommy. I'm afraid you're fare won't be coming with you. We'll be looking after him. On your way now. I might need to speak to you later, but no worries for you". Then I turned and walked away. Tommy was halfway down Ralph Allen Drive before he came to enough to realise he had not called in that he had lost the fare and was available for another job.

I climbed into the back of the car beside Tom Stevens, who sat upright, looking straight forward, but totally unseeingly. He showed no emotion.

"Right, Deek. Out of here."

"What about his luggage?"

"Leave it! It'll be safer not to touch it. What do you say, Mr. Stevens?" There was no reply, nor recognition of hearing the question.

"Just get us out of here. Block off the end of the road. Then call in that we have taken into custody a man on suspicion of last night's bomb attack. We'll need all services up here, now. Especially the bomb squad. Maybe the boss has got things moving, but call in anyway".

Deek almost did not make it through the gateway. Suddenly his palms were very sweaty, and slippery on the driving wheel.

57

"What did you think you were doing? I told you to go home! Are you sick, or something?" The incongruity of the question was lost on the person posing it. D.I. Welsh had been working himself into a lather for the best part of an hour, since he had taken the call from the mobile 'phone.

Friday evening in Bath was bad at any time. On the night of the Festival opening it was worse with all those coming into town for the event. On such a night with a main street still closed off it was claustrophobic. It was hell on four wheels. Even with emergency lights flashing those that needed to get to Combe Down had made little progress by the time the call from the Deek came in.

Now he was facing my ghostly countenance, that of the man who had saved the city's name and festival by finding the bomber. The festival could go ahead, not that I was aware of that, or had it foremost in my mind. He may have been glad we had the bomber but he was more than upset my actions and not telling what was going on, and for looking like death itself.

"Why didn't you tell me what was going on?"

"Boss, I tried."

"Not much you did. Did you know when I sent you home?"

My grey face took on an even more pained expression, as my mind tried to fathom an answer. "I kind of thought, but didn't know for sure, or who".

My body started to fold as my knees gave up on the strength to hold it up any longer. Ian Welsh grabbed his me by the lapels, holding me up. For the first time that day I could sense him relax. "Got to give you credit. However you did it, it was good work".

I allowed myself a little smile at that thought. Ian

did not lack just that little compassion, despite his background.

58

Five minutes before six o'clock the Deputy Chief Constable was stepping out of his car as the radio crackled into life.

The day had been long and frustrating. Absolutely no breakthrough had been reported in the investigation. The City Fathers would not like what he had to say, but there was no backing down this time. The concert would not go on, even though nothing suspicious had been found on the ground.

His thoughts were interrupted by his driver. "Sir, this call is for you. It seems important." He listened intently to the message, giving his confirmation at intervals. At its end he sighed deeply and gathered himself before striding towards his meeting.

Once again he was met by seven pairs of eyes as he entered the room. Again those eyes conveyed apprehension, a little hope and a lot of questioning.

"Good evening, everyone. It might not be quite six o'clock but I see no point in keeping you waiting..."

There was an intake of breath from those in the room. Eyelids closed to fend off the next word.

"...you may have the concert. We have the bomber."

The hallelujahs echoed around the room in the rejoicing.

59

Things changed, but stayed the same. As the consultant, Dr. Knightley was a constant. So was Sister Gillen. The nursing staff rotated, always re-appearing.

After only two months of my treatment Emily disappeared to a new position in London. Her replacement was a bright, energetic young man called Peter who had moved from a hospital in Plymouth.

Following the fourth intrathecal injection Harry left. By then I had become very confident that I was not going to be consigned to a wheel chair. I knew the pattern of how to lie in the foetal position so that Harry could feel down the nodules of my spine to find the right space to insert the needle. It was no longer a concern.

The fifth month was different. It was so very different.

Peter had assumed Harry's role. The warming up exercises of feeling up and down the spine was exactly as Harry had always done. The insertion of the needle did not feel as free as before. Suddenly I felt a shock, as an electric current, shoot down my right leg. The needle was withdrawn.

Several other attempts were made with equal lack of success, but with variations on the shocks travelling through my body. More and more I began to appreciate what electrical torture would be like. The needle was not going in where it should. Nerves were being hit. Reaction was beginning to wrack my body. I could feel apprehension, and a little perspiration was gathering on my brow.

The increasing laboured breathing and muttered

apologies from behind me indicated Peter was becoming equally anxious. In the end he called a halt.

"Sorry. I'm going to stop. I'm not getting this right today. I'm going to get help. Vinjay started last week. He's had lots of experience doing this. I'll get him to try."

Five minutes later Vinjay successfully slid the home at the first attempt. It was one disc lower than where Peter had been trying.

Relief was palpable all round. Success did not always come easily. It had to be worked for. I thought that pretty well summed up the whole cancer care situation.

60

"We have some breaking news. Scotland Yard has just announced that a man has been arrested for the bombing incident at Bath Railway station yesterday evening.

No details have yet been released but it does seem that no one else is thought to be involved.

The time is now 6.15."

61

The opening concert to the Festival seemed to go with extra vitality. The music seemed more magical, more tuned than ever before. The applause was more rapturous than on any previous year. There was a groundswell of sheer relief and vitality from everyone there.

By the time of the finale, and accompanying firework display, the man whose detective work ensured it could all go ahead was in bed, fast asleep. Getting home had been a blur. I knew I had been driven home. Whether by taxi, or police car, I could not remember. Whichever it was I was sure I had not paid for it. I came to myself standing in the kitchen.

Normally, after a success I would have enjoyed a celebratory drink. Not tonight. There would be no pints drunk, no whisky, and certainly no champagne. Instead I celebrated by finishing off the last night's baked beans with a glass of water. I did not have the energy, or inclination, to hang around to even make a hot drink.

I stumbled to bed and quickly surrendered consciousness. By ten o'clock I was sleeping the sleep of the good, as well as that of the nearly dead.

62

The forces dressed in black were sweeping all before them. Individually they had no form. The black was not of colour, but of intent. It was bad. It was evil. It was destructive.

The opposition was uncomprehending. There was no recognition of the dark intent of the force before it. The black tide swept on. The good, the well intentioned, the righteous, were being trampled. The opposition was being overpowered because the only weapons it was using were appeasement, compromise and complacency.

The forces in black had no fear of appeasement. In fact they loved it. It gave them more time to manoeuvre into better positions to strike further. They had no truck with compromise. They saw that only as a licence to probe further. Compromise represented weakness. It represented ineffectiveness. It allowed an opportunity to take control. It allowed an opportunity to win.

Complacency comforted the uncommitted and indifferent. There was no need to take a stand against anything. There was no desire to be involved in making decisions. Things were fine. Things would always be fine. There was no inclination towards anything else. So complacency slept the slumber of the contented while the black forces eroded the areas around it.

The black force was overcoming my body. I could see how the cancer had burst forth in my body even if I could not understand how it had seen the opportunity to attack.

In my mind I saw the grainy black and white film of Neville Chamberlain waving a piece of paper, only to be followed by pictures of the Panzer divisions sweeping into Poland. I saw the young ned smirking at being sentenced to 120 hours community service after beating a complete stranger so badly he lost the sight in one eye.

I saw the man in the black coat and scythe directing his supporters to stifle the life out of me. I saw the darkness sweeping over life itself.

Then I felt the uplift that came from the chemotherapy. A decision had been made to fight back. I felt the power that came from positive resolve return. I felt the black forces being repelled until they were forced back into containment. I knew it was happening. I felt the fighting in my body. It was no easy fight. The collateral damage was immense. There would be a massive rebuilding programme, but it would be achieved. I had not surrendered.

The dreams had not stopped just because I was clear of the treatment. As I lay in my bed I saw all of it through the torment of my sleep. However, I did not see the same resolve in society as I had tried to keep through all those months of treatment. Rather I saw the apologists and rights activists leading society into a spiral of degeneration, and the silent majority following like sheep.

63

The firework display exploded over the Bath skies. Each bang and whoosh indicated another panoply of colour and design.

In his cell Tom heard each one but nothing registered. He stared in front of him oblivious to all around him. The past four hours had been a void. The days and weeks ahead would be the same. There was no future to look forward to and in his mind there was no achievement to his latest aim. There was no salve to his destiny.

There had been questions but he had not responded. The family solicitor had appeared at some point but he had not acknowledged him.

He sat on the cot, an empty shell, with no shred of guilt, remorse, or life.

64

"So, what's to happen now? Are we going to see justice?" Jimsi asked the questions as he placed the two glasses on the table.

We were sitting at an outside table of the "George" pub, beside the canal at Bathampton. It was a popular drinking hole for canal walkers, canal boat users, and the well appointed local clientele. It was an old pub of considerable character with low, beamed ceilings.

We had come down the hill in the bright sunshine for a late lunchtime drink. The main crowd had moved on so they had the luxury of a table to ourselves. There was just the nagging doubt about being able to get back up the hill in good order.

I placed my hands around the base of my pint feeling the cool dampness of the condensation forming on the glass. From under the brim of my hat, that I still wore to protect my head, I looked through the golden hue of my lager shandy. Two weeks after my first thought of having a drink, here it was, at last.

The exertions of that weekend had proved too much for me. My body had lost too much strength to stand what had been demanded of it during the chase. Even worse had been the time spent report writing afterwards.

"Doubt it ", I eventually replied. " By the time the case is ready for court he'll probably be dead. If he's not, he's not likely to be in a fit condition to plead. "

"But why did he do it? It's hard to say. Rottenness, pain, jealousy, anger. He was - is - a young lad. Had everything going for him. Looks, career prospects, money, women. Then he saw the door being slammed shut. He got cancer. Melanoma, skin cancer. There's been lots about it in the papers in recent times. They've almost made it the new designer cancer to have. No way out for him as it was diagnosed very late. His fault for not checking it out sooner. He thought it was totally unfair. Just couldn't accept it should happen to him. Sure, he thought he was special, and it should only happen to plebs who weren't him. Couldn't get his head round that cancer isn't fair. Couldn't accept that it takes people in so many different ways. He got the worst hand. Couldn't accept that. All he saw for his life could be taken away so quickly. Couldn't accept that others would just go on living. So he wanted a revenge before he went. He just decided to take as many with him as he could. Maybe it was his last throw at being top dog. He made the rules. He placed the stakes. He was in charge.

In many ways he was unlucky getting caught. We were lucky. How would we have unravelled it? No Al Quaeda. No animal rights movement. No one else claiming responsibility. No previous intelligence. Nothing. No message. No clues. "

"Just you going to Willie Budd's at the same time! Must have been some sort of fate. Written in the stars. More like the depths of hell", was Jimsi's response.

"You know, Jimsi, when this all started with me I sort of thought cancer was a corruption of a cell that tainted those around it. You know, like one misguided idiot being lead down the path of evil and convincing a few others the world would only be a better place if they killed off "the establishment". But it's not like that at all. Cancer is always there. We always have bad cells - cancer cells - in our bodies. Normally the good cells, the good guys, keep them in check. It's only when the good cells weaken, or are distracted, that the baddies burst out and show themselves as what we call cancer. A bit like when the veneer of civilised living slips. A bit like crime. Always there. But as long as there are strong laws, sound enforcement and so on it is kept in check. Weaken the resolve and you have a crime wave. Never thought of cancer as a comparison to civilisation".

Jimsi looked at me reflectively. I could see what he was thinking. I knew what he was going to say. We had known each other too long not to. "You're a good boy. You stood up to everything well. Never downbeat. Always positive; up for the fight, you always said it was the only way to be". We both remembered someone from years ago who just lain down and waited to die when he had been diagnosed. No, I had not done that. I had come through with the help of medical advances, the dedication of those caring for me, support of friends and family, but equally by my own determination.

True, I still had the radiotherapy on my remaining testicle to go through, but that was just a safeguard. It would be a mild experience in comparison, even if it would finally kill off any prospects of me ever becoming a father.

My story would only ever be my story, but there were many others who could tell comparable tales of seeing off the "Big C". It was unfortunate that there were too many who would not have the opportunity.

"Well, it's good you stuck with it. It's good to have you still with us. Here's to you. Cheers!"

As I raised my glass in response to Jimsi's toast the light struck the side of it. It was a quick flash, just as quick as a cobra striking.

65

Tom Stevens never did go to trial. From the moment he was arrested the fire and anger inside was extinguished. The cancer in his mind died leaving no fight, no desire, no will. He gave in to what he had known was inevitable, but the drive for revenge had been denied him. So he was left with nothing.

The cancer in his body took longer to achieve his end, but that was just three months.

Before he died his parents had sold the house and moved away. They came to visit him but there was no bond with him. Neither was there between them. Both had retired into their own world. Both felt confusion, despair and loss over what had become of their son, and how he had discredited them. Both felt the loss of their status and standing brought about by their new notoriety. Neither could come to terms with what had happened. Neither had the strength to support the other. In time they would drift apart altogether.

So Tom did achieve some form of return for his campaign of retribution. He destroyed the lives of his mother and father, ended three lives at bath Spa Station, and caused anguish to their families and friends and left those who survived with varying degrees of injury and trauma for a long time to come.

There was no happy ending for any of them.

66

Two years later the cancer returned. The fight was on again.

As I absorbed the news it conjured renewed images. Again I saw the correlation between crime and cancer. Both were always there. Both always seemed to be looking for a way to break out. Both needed to be closely watched. There was no scope to take a relaxed attitude to either.

During those two years I had been back to the hospital regularly for checks on my condition. I had seen Karen on more than a few occasions and any damage to our relationship had long since been repaired, if not taken any further. Now I would be back for longer periods again for more treatment. Maybe, just maybe, now that the cycle had turned, I would summon up the nerve to invite her to take a run out with me and Miss Daisy sometime.

There is a popular belief that in everything there is a beginning, a middle, and an end. What is not necessarily understood is where the parameters of each stage transfer. In life is beginning the birth? Or is it the moment of conception? Or is it the moment of desire awakening that will cause the conception? Or is it the births of the children that will give rise to the next generation of births? As to death is that the end , or is it another beginning?

I have no answers. Neither to those questions, nor why I was struck by Lymphoma. Just as no one else can tell me why I became so fated, nor why so many others are struck by other forms of cancer.

Dear Reader,

I hope you enjoyed your reading of the book. It is dedicated to all those who work to relieve the pain and stress caused through cancer. That ranges from those undertaking research to all those involved in frontline care. The idea of writing the book came during my first encounter with cancer. I was diagnosed with lymphoma in the spring of 2005 and treated on William Budd Ward, Royal United Hospital, Bath. To those who may have wondered, it really does exist.

At the time I thought that was going to be the extent of my experiences. However that has not been the case. I have now been diagnosed four times finishing my last round of treatment in April this year. Towards the end of my six months chemotherapy in Bath we moved to North Lincolnshire, and now I have reason to be grateful for the support I have had from Scunthorpe General Hospital, Lincoln County Hospital and Castle Hill Hospital, Hull.

Whilst I am grateful to everyone, and they are too numerous to mention, there are those that need to be specially recognised. At Bath, in Dr. Knechtli's team there was registrar Dr. Masurekar, better known as Ash, and a cancer care dynamo in the form of Sister Caroline Gilleece. I have heard she is now a matron – and well worth it she is!

At Lincoln Dr. Sheehan's team have taken me through courses of radiotherapy three times. The last time I saw him for a consultation he seemed past the stage of being surprised to see me again.

In 2009 I had a stem cell transplant at Castle Hill Hospital, Hull. The three week treatment was the most demanding experience I have endured but Dr. Russell Patmore, and his team, saw me through. Any untoward experience I may have avoided previously caught up with me then. Even that did not see the end of it and it came back again.

They only team left to be recognised is that at Scunthorpe General Hospital. Since I moved to this part of the country I have been looked after by Dr. Sanjeev Jalahal, who has watched over me like a guardian angel, and Clinical Nurse Specialist Helen Carolan. They provide me with support and give me total confidence with their care and attention.

In the story all the account, and thoughts, of cancer and its treatments are mine. They are as close to factual recollection as I can muster from medical records, memory and reminiscences with others. Equally the rest of the story line is pure fiction.

The characters, as portrayed, do not exist. However many do have alter egos in real life. Names, descriptions, characteristics have been changed to suit the story. All are intended as statements of appreciation and the first adaptations to be acknowledged are Dr. Knetchli (Dr. Knightly), Caroline Gilleece (Karen) and Ash (Harry).

Outside of the medial characters Jimsi and Niki are unashamedly based on my old friends Jamie and Nicky Garden. If the truth be told, other than the name chance, Jimsi is Jamie.

Bob Smith is an appreciation of Bill Steele. I first met Bill in 1966 (!) when we worked together in Perth. My last post in the Ministry of Defence was taking over Bill when he retired. After that he became a friend of RUH Bath, joining his wife, Anne, in that voluntary work. Bill did serve me tea in William Budd, and he did do the investigation into its name, Anne was an early critic of my writing. My thanks, and appreciations go to both.

Two retired senior police officers, Ken Bates and Ian Welch, now both working for Lincolnshire Safer Neighbourhoods Partnership, helped me with points on police aspects. Ian had no objections to me adapting his name.

Another mention has to go to Jamie – how he will love being the most often mentioned – for his notes on the Command Structure.

Other thanks for factual aspects go to my elder son, Donald. Among his loves are engineering and cars, not inherited from me, and he provided the background to create Miss Daisy.

Also my elder step-son, Neil, provided me with help on the background for the Japanese girls. Neil now lives in Baltimore, Maryland with his American wife, Allison, who he met while they were both teaching English in Japan.

Thanks go to my friend and neighbour, Paul Vernum, for providing the artistic input to the cover design, and to all those who have read the drafts and commented. That particularly applies to James Laurenson, actor and near neighbour when we lived in Somerset, who when I expressed doubts over having the ability and energy to get beyond the concept stage told me it was my idea, and I should do it. Also as my typing is strictly of a slow, slow, slower tempo I am grateful to a young lady called Emily Colecchia, for doing my retyping. I must also add thanks to Brad Jacobs for taking the photograph shown on the back cover, one we both truly love.

It would be entirely remiss of me not to recognise the support of all my immediate family, extended family and friends, with special mention for Rod and Sue Poustie, for their support over the past turbulent years. I struggled to think of a title for the book and it was during a conversation Sue used the expression that caught my attention, and solved the problem.

I have always had a sounding board in my little sister, and nurse, Rhoda, which has helped keep me stable. Also, my other sister, Rosilyn, for her intuitive suggestion of the biblical reference.

Lastly I come to the person who has been with me and seen me through it all, my wife, Katherine. She has endured it all, which is particularly ironic as I took early retirement to help her through poor health. I have admitted to myself to having a few bad tempered days during the treatment. If the truth be told there have been a lot more than I would wish to acknowledge but she has stuck by and loved me anyway.

So, having hopefully enjoyed the read I would like to think you will support me with one last thought. In buying this book you have helped make a financial contribution to Cancer Research UK and the Lymphoma Association for the work they do. My sincere thanks for that.

Best wishes and good health to you.

Ron Stewart

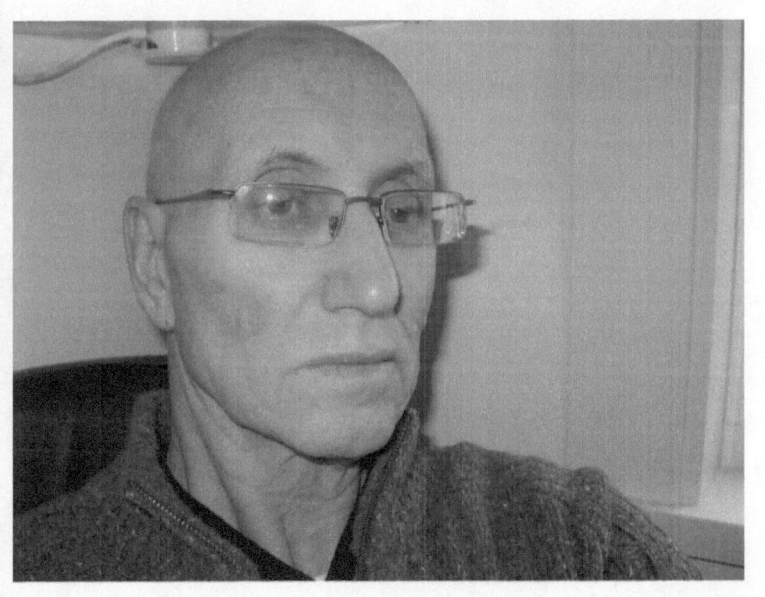

Ron after treatment, February 2009.